Dedications

To our families for their unyielding love and support and to those personally and professionally known, who have inspired our passion to improve recognition of and response to resuscitation emergencies.

Practical Resuscitation for Healthcare Professionals

SECOND EDITION

EDITED BY

Pam Moule
RN, DipN, DipNE, BSc (Hons), MSc, EdD
Reader in Nursing and Learning Technologies
University of the West of England,
Bristol

AND

John W. Albarran
RN, DipN (Lon.), BSc (Hons), PG Dip Ed, MSc, DPhil NFESC
Reader in Critical Care Nursing
University of the West of England,
Bristol

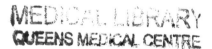

WILEY-BLACKWELL

A John Wiley & Sons, Ltd., Publication

This edition first published 2009
© 2009 by Blackwell Publishing Ltd

Blackwell Publishing was acquired by John Wiley & Sons in February 2007. Blackwell's publishing programme has been merged with Wiley's global Scientific, Technical, and Medical business to form Wiley-Blackwell.

Registered office
John Wiley & Sons Ltd, The Atrium, Southern Gate, Chichester, West Sussex, PO19 8SQ, United Kingdom

Editorial offices
9600 Garsington Road, Oxford, OX4 2DQ, United Kingdom
350 Main Street, Malden, MA 02148-5020, USA

1006193945

For details of our global editorial offices, for customer services and for information about how to apply for permission to reuse the copyright material in this book please see our website at www.wiley.com/wiley-blackwell.

The right of the author to be identified as the author of this work has been asserted in accordance with the Copyright, Designs and Patents Act 1988.

Library of Congress Cataloging-in-Publication Data

Practical resuscitation for healthcare professionals / edited by Pam Moule and John W. Albarran. – 2nd ed.
      p. ; cm.
   Rev. ed. of: Practical resuscitation : recognition and response / edited by Pam Moule and John W. Albarran. c2005.
   Includes bibliographical references and index.
   ISBN 978-1-4051-9354-2 (pbk. : alk. paper)   1. Resuscitation.   2. Emergency nursing.
I. Moule, Pam.   II. Albarran, John W.   III. Practical resuscitation.
   [DNLM: 1. Resuscitation–methods. 2. Emergency Treatment–methods. WA 292 P895 2009]
   RC87.9.P73 2009
   616.02′5–dc22   2008044707

A catalogue record for this book is available from the British Library.

Set in 10/12 pt Palatino by Aptara® Inc., New Delhi, India
Printed and bound in Malaysia by KHL Printing Co Sdn Bhd

1   2009

Contents

Foreword

In the UK in 2005, heart disease was the leading cause of death in males and females, accounting for one in five and one in six deaths, respectively, and at an average age of 68 for men and 73 for women. The incidence of out-of-hospital cardiac arrest in England is approximately 113/100 000 population per annum. The only effective management of a cardiac arrest in any setting is the swift response of a knowledgeable and well-rehearsed team.

Clearly, then, the development and maintenance of effective resuscitation skills is essential in all health care workers working in acute settings. Despite this unarguable fact there is a wealth of evidence to suggest that both basic and advanced cardiopulmonary resuscitation knowledge and skills are both poorly acquired and poorly retained (even over intervals of a few months) regardless of the grade or profession of health care practitioners. It is worth remembering that the main responsibility for ensuring competence lies with each individual registered practitioner.

Practical resuscitation for healthcare professionals provides practitioners with a valuable aid to acquire and maintain the underpinning knowledge necessary for the safe and effective performance of the full gamut of resuscitation skills. It has a concise and clear writing style which means that it can be read from cover to cover in a matter of a few hours, but its structured chapters also support its use as a reference or revision text for the more experienced professional.

It is written and edited by a small team of educators and researchers with experience and broad knowledge of their subject matter. Their evidence-based approach to the topic is underpinned by a large number of references which permit readers to further explore any area of particular interest. Each chapter is presented in a consistent manner, including clear aims and learning outcomes and ending with a review of key learning points, and a case study to allow the reader to self-test their knowledge. Appropriate guidelines are cited and reproduced and the use of photographs, algorithms and key actions presented as bullet points all add to the clarity and readability of the text. The editors have wisely included separate chapters on areas of resuscitation known to be of particular concern to non-specialist healthcare professionals, including ethics, paediatrics, the management of reversible causes of cardiac arrest and the management of cardiac arrest in special circumstances.

This book will be of considerable value to all healthcare providers, regardless of their level of seniority and experience and of their discipline and professional group. More importantly, if studied thoroughly it has the potential to be of considerably greater value to their patients.

Prof. Malcolm Woollard, MPH, MBA, MA(Ed), Dip IMC (RCSEd),
PGCE, RN, SRPara, NFESC, FASI, FHEA, FACAP

Professor in Pre-hospital and Emergency Care & Director,
Pre-hospital, Emergency & Cardiovascular Care
Applied Research Group, Coventry University

Honorary Consultant Paramedic, West Midlands & South
East Coast Ambulance Service NHS Trusts

Professor in Pre-hospital Care,
Charles Sturt University (NSW, Australia)

Honorary Senior Research Fellow,
Monash University (Victoria, Australia)

Preface

This second edition reflects changes in resuscitation guidelines published in 2005. The field of resuscitation is an area where theory and practice continue to develop at a very rapid pace. Advances in technology and an increase in the number of published quality research papers mean that guidelines are revised periodically so that standards in cardiopulmonary resuscitation can reflect the most current thinking and application of technical skills. The increased patient dependency, now common within many hospital and community settings, has further emphasised the need for healthcare professionals to become competent in basic life support and, increasingly, immediate life support skills.

The premise behind this book is that healthcare professionals starting their career as practitioners need to be equipped with a blend of theoretical and practice-based skills in order to be effective as first responders, resuscitation team members or leaders of the arrest situation. This textbook therefore approaches knowledge and skill development in resuscitation from a practical viewpoint and includes the underpinning current evidence base to support resuscitation skill delivery.

The book includes key chapters presenting the main resuscitation algorithms and this second edition includes a new chapter on Paediatric Life Support (Chapter 8). All the updated chapters present the current evidence base for practice presented in a format that we hope will be accessible to the novice and informative for those staff more experienced in resuscitation.

There is no doubt that the first experience of participating in an arrest is terrifying, whatever the role or activity adopted. We expect the reader will become more confident and proficient in assessing, responding to and reviewing resuscitation situations. Moreover, we hope that this textbook will stimulate greater interest and enthusiasm in the resuscitation field.

Pam Moule and John W. Albarran

Acknowledgements

The editors are grateful to the following staff from the University of the West of England, Bristol:

- Dave Watkins, Senior Skills Technician; and Neil Wakeman, Skills Technician, for their assistance with photographs;
- Jane Wathen, Graphic Designer, for help with some of the images;
- To a number of colleagues who kindly gave their time and agreed to pose for the photographs in this textbook.

We also owe thanks to:

- Resuscitation Council UK for permission to use resuscitation algorithms in a number of chapters;
- British Medical Association for permission to use the decision-making framework, decisions relating to cardiopulmonary resuscitation, in Chapter 2;
- Connect Publishing Limited for permission to use family witnessed resuscitation position statement in Chapter 2;
- Laerdal® for permission to use the change of survival image in Chapter 5.

Contributors

John W. Albarran
Reader in Critical Care Nursing, University of the West of England, Bristol

Rebecca Hoskins
Nurse Consultant in Emergency Care, University Hospitals Bristol NHS
Foundation Trust and University of the West of England, Bristol

Ben King
Senior Resuscitation Officer, Gloucestershire Royal Hospital, Gloucester

Una McKay
Clinical Skills Demonstrator, University of the West of England, Bristol

Pam Moule
Reader in Nursing and Learning Technologies, University of the West of
England, Bristol

Paul Snelling
Senior Lecturer, University of the West of England, Gloucestershire

Jas Soar
Consultant in Anaesthesia and Intensive Care Medicine, Southmead Hospital,
Bristol

Jackie Younker
Senior Lecturer, University of the West of England, Bristol

Section 1

Introduction and Professional Issues

1 | Resuscitation Policy and Educational Developments

Pam Moule & John W. Albarran

INTRODUCTION

Resuscitation is relatively new to the world of evidence-based practice, being founded on a limited, but increasing body of scientific evidence as the basis for current best practice. International collaboration and consensus has also been instrumental to the development of resuscitation guidelines that seek to standardise the management approach of cardiac arrests and other life-threatening conditions for both adults and children. This chapter explores the current policy and trends in resuscitation education and training. The chapter concludes with a guide to the book's contents and its use.

AIMS

This chapter outlines the current policy position and reviews the importance of educational preparation in developing knowledge and skills in resuscitation. In addition, it intends to prepare readers to use the remainder of the book.

LEARNING OUTCOMES

By the end of the chapter, the reader will be able to:

❏ identify the current policy informing resuscitation guidelines;
❏ examine competency debates in the field and current trends in educational preparation for resuscitation;
❏ demonstrate how to use this book.

CURRENT POLICY

Following the introduction of modern cardiopulmonary resuscitation (CPR) nearly 50 years ago (American Heart Association (AHA) and International Liaison Committee on Resuscitation (ILCOR) 2000a), guidelines for the delivery of basic life support (BLS) and advanced life support (ALS) have been through a period of evolutionary change. Guidelines produced in 2000 (AHA and ILCOR 2000b) were the culmination of wide international collaboration. They aimed to achieve internationally accepted, comprehensive, evidence-based guides for resuscitation practice, and included paediatric and adult BLS and ALS algorithms.

Wider acceptance of standardised, evidence-based approaches to resuscitation has aimed to reduce and simplify the number of skills required to enable the lay public and health professionals to respond promptly and effectively. Indeed, resuscitation teams are more likely to function with some coherency and expertise, as elements of inconsistency in practice are removed.

As with previous recommendations and policy statements, the introduction of the 2005 Resuscitation guidelines sought to reflect a consensus of science and emphasised the need for continued updating and revision (Nolan 2006). Through standardisation, it has been possible to simplify procedures, supporting ease of skill and knowledge development and retention. This simplification has been afforded through the critical appraisal of available scientific evidence, a base that is set to continue to inform the ongoing development of resuscitation care as new scientific findings emerge. To achieve consensus, all resuscitation councils and experts employed a systematic approach to developing the evidence base.

The current guidelines are based on the 2005 International Consensus on Cardiopulmonary Resuscitation and Emergency Cardiovascular Care Science with Treatment, Recommendations (CoSTR). The European Resuscitation Council (ERC) Guidelines (2005) are derived from the CoSTR document but reflect the European context and practice. The ERC Executive Committee in recommending guidelines anticipates local, regional and national adaptations that reflect the availability of drugs, equipment and human resources.

Demographics on in-hospital and out-of-hospital cardiac arrests suggest the continuing need for professionals and members of the lay public to engage with resuscitation. To enhance the best outcomes of resuscitation, those responding to cardiac arrests must be in possession of the necessary knowledge and skills to perform timely, safe and effective resuscitation.

Challenges in developing competent responders
BLS is a formalised component of the competency framework for registered professionals. This suggests an assumed need for competency in BLS as part of the professional's repertoire of skills.

Competency-based curricula identify the knowledge and skills that a professional is expected to possess on qualification or completion of course, for members of the public. It reflects a current political ideology that attempts to remove the potential risk to society from any nurse or other professional delivering CPR. The current preoccupation with risk emanates from ambivalence about the expertise of professionals in performing their duties. This concern is fuelled by recent evidence of professional incompetence and malpractice presented in the media and has supported a series of measures to increase professional scrutiny and accountability, which includes competency development.

Knowledge and skill acquisition and retention are requirements of competency development and maintenance. Resuscitation teaching and ongoing practice development, requiring sustained educational commitment of practitioners to maintain competence, supports competency development (Baskett et al. 2005).

There are many challenges in maintaining competency for individuals and employing organisations. Despite a long tradition in CPR training, there remain a number of unresolved issues with achieving competency and retention of skills. Studies suggest that course delivery is not always effective in the promotion of CPR skills (Perkins et al. 2008, Verplancke et al. 2008). The barriers to skill acquisition are also attributed to long training intervals and lack of feedback on technique (Abella *et al.* 2007).

Consequently, the Resuscitation Councils and others have engaged in the development and evaluation of training curricula to support recommendations of educational programmes which optimise the acquisition and retention of knowledge and skills by a range of providers (Beckers *et al.* 2005, Harve & Silvfast 2004, Hoke *et al.* 2006, Priori *et al.* 2004). Most approaches adopt the principles of adult education and learning to underpin training. These include small group facilitation with interactive discussion and hands-on practice (Baskett 2004). The ratio of instructors is recommended as 1:3 to 1:6. It is also suggested that core knowledge should be made available prior to practice and assessment of skills (Baskett *et al.* 2005). A number of delivery modes exist, including video instruction, Power-Point presentations, CD-ROMs and online learning materials (Moule & Albarran 2002). As training aims to develop and sustain competence, it is recommended that a test of core knowledge should be included with an assessment of practical skills and scenario management (Baskett *et al.* 2005). A number of sophisticated simulation and virtual reality techniques can support this (Chamberlain & Hazinski 2003). The use of simulation and assessment through objective structured clinical examinations (OSCEs) allows the rehearsal of resuscitation skills amongst interprofessional groups and provides opportunities for feedback and learning (Moule *et al.* 2008). Peer assessment can form part of the learning process, being used successfully in the development of BLS skills in undergraduate training (Bucknall *et al.* 2008).

Resuscitation skill development should be supported by appropriately trained professionals who have complete relevant and specific preparation (Baskett *et al.* 2005). Instructors should adopt a supportive role in delivery and testing to ensure competence.

HOW TO USE THIS BOOK
This book is underpinned by a philosophy that embraces the wider view of resuscitation presented in the above discussion. The text emphasises the importance of recognising and responding to critical care needs within both the community and hospital settings. It hopes to support healthcare workers in developing the knowledge and skills required to operate effectively in an environment that requires them to both recognise and respond to deteriorating conditions.

Structure and content
This book contains 17 chapters, written by experts in their area, that inform and develop through the provision of evidence-based guidance, supporting questioning and enhancement of clinical competencies in practice delivery. Every chapter is presented in an accessible manner, using a structured format:

- Introduction – is an overview of the chapter content.
- Aims – guide the reader to the key aims of the chapter, enabling selective and appropriate reading.
- Learning outcomes – identify the key learning for the reader.

- Content (guidelines, evidence-based literature, steps in the skill) – provides the reader with the knowledge development and evidence base, stressing practice skill delivery.
- Review of key learning points – provides a useful and concise resume of key learning for the reader.
- Case studies – offer an opportunity for readers to test their understanding and development of the key issues presented in the chapter.
- Reference lists – provide the reader with an opportunity to further explore reference material and develop wider reading.

Practical use

Whilst the book can be consumed in its entirety, it supports selective use in the practice setting, to facilitate effective recognition and response to cardiac arrest events. The structure and content of the book should be used as a guide to identifying specific learning opportunities that can be matched to individual learning needs. In this way, maximum benefit can be gained from the book.

The evidence base presented will support care delivery, whilst key skill delivery, presented through a step-by-step approach, should enhance confidence and competence development. Review of learning within chapters facilitates readers to be aware of the fundamental practice principles.

Where presented, the case study examples provide scope to test individual understanding of the evidence base and steps in skill delivery. Learning can be further enhanced through exploration of the reference material provided.

CONCLUSIONS

This chapter considers the current policy context and educational developments in resuscitation. As a result of ongoing scientific advances in resuscitation, health professionals must remain updated to ensure that they are competent in both preventing and managing cardiac arrests. There also remain a number of challenges to optimising standardised skill acquisition and maintenance in evolving discipline. Innovative, student-orientated and interactive modes of learning that emphasise feedback on performance are one way forward. In addition, opportunities for skill rehearsal through simulation or virtual environments can assist with this endeavour.

This textbook aims to present a comprehensive of the current evidence base of resuscitation in a practical and accessible way that will enable readers to further develop their expertise in this area of professional practice.

REFERENCES

Abella, B.S., Edelson, D.P., Kim, S. *et al.* (2007) CPR quality improvement during in-hospital cardiac arrest using a real-dash time audio visual feedback system. *Resuscitation* **73**, 54–61.

American Heart Association and International Liaison Committee on Resuscitation (2000a) Part 1. Introduction to the International Guidelines 2000 for CPR and ECC. A consensus on science. *Resuscitation* **46**, 3–15.

American Heart Association and International Liaison Committee on Resuscitation (2000b) Part 3. Adult basic life support. *Resuscitation* **46**, 29–71.

Baskett, P. (2004) Progress of the advanced life support courses in Europe and beyond. *Resuscitation* **62**, 311–13.

Baskett, P.J.F., Nolan, J.P., Handley, A., Soar, J., Biarent, D. & Richmond, S. (2005) European Resuscitation Council guidelines for resuscitation 2005. Section 9: principles of training in resuscitation. *Resuscitation* **67** (suppl 1), S181–9.

Beckers, S., Fries, M., Bickenbach, J., Derwall, M., Kuhlen, R. & Rossaint, R. (2005) Minimal instructions improve the performance of laypersons in the use of semi-automatic and automatic external defibrillators. *Critical Care Forum* **9** (2), R110–16. Available online at: http://ccforum.com/content/9/2/R110.

Bucknall, V., Sobic, E.M., Wood, H.L., Howlett, S.C., Taylor, R. & Perkins, G.D. (2008) Peer assessment of resuscitation skills. *Resuscitation* **77**, 211–15.

Chamberlain, D.A. & Hazinski, N.F. (2003) Education in resuscitation. *Resuscitation* **59**, 11–43.

European Resuscitation Council (2005) European Resuscitation Council guidelines for resuscitation 2005. *Resuscitation* **67** (suppl 1), S7–23, S25–37.

Harve, H. & Silfvast, T. (2004) The use of automated external defibrillators by non-medical first responders in Finland. *European Journal of Emergency Medicine* **11** (3), 130–33.

Hoke, R., Chamberlain, D. & Handley, A. (2006) A reference automated external defibrillator provider course for Europe. *Resuscitation* **69** (3), 421–33.

Moule, P. & Albarran, J.W. (2002) Automated external defibrillation as part of BLS: implications for education and practice. *Resuscitation* **54**, 223–30.

Moule, P., Albarran, J.W., Bessant, E., Brownfield, C. & Pollock, J. (2008) A non-randomised comparison of e-learning and classroom delivery of basic life support with automated external defibrillator use: a pilot study. *International Journal of Nursing Practice* **14**, 425–32.

Nolan, JP. (2006) Introduction. In: Baskett, P. & Nolan, J. (eds) *A Pocket Book of the European Resuscitation Council Guidelines for Resuscitation 2005*. Mosby-Elsevier, Edinburgh.

Perkins, G.D., Boyle, W., Bridgestock, H. *et al.* (2008) Quality of CPR during advanced resuscitation training. *Resuscitation* **77**, 69–74.

Priori, S.G., Bossaert, L., Chamberlain, D.A. *et al.* (2004) ESC-ERC recommendations for the use of automated external defibrillators (AEDs) in Europe. *European Heart Journal* **25** (5), 437–45.

Verplancke, T., Paepe, P.D., Calle, P.A. *et al.* (2008) Determinants of the quality of basic life support by hospital nurses. *Resuscitation* **77**, 75–80.

Professional, Ethical and Legal Issues | 2

John W. Albarran & Paul Snelling

INTRODUCTION

International collaboration has supported the development of resuscitation guidelines that seek to provide a consensus view for practice. This chapter outlines major ethical, professional and legal issues surrounding resuscitation and presents roles and responsibilities of the 'first responder' in an emergency arrest situation.

AIMS

This chapter introduces professional issues in resuscitation and gives an overview of the roles of healthcare professionals in a resuscitation attempt.

LEARNING OUTCOMES

By the end of the chapter, the reader will be able to:

❏ discuss the ethical and legal implications of *do not attempt resuscitation orders*;
❏ explore the debates related to the *presence of family members* during resuscitation;
❏ examine the ethical dilemmas associated with deciding *when to discontinue resuscitation attempts*;
❏ appreciate the *different roles of cardiac arrest team members* and how to work with the team.

'DO NOT ATTEMPT RESUSCITATION' ORDERS

In 2007, the Royal College of Nursing (RCN), the Resuscitation Council (UK) and the British Medical Association (BMA) jointly published *Decisions Relating to Cardiopulmonary Resuscitation*. This document is freely available via the internet (Resuscitation Council UK 2007), and should be regarded as required reading for anybody involved in resuscitation. The decision-making framework from this document is reprinted here as Figure 2.1. Decisions not to attempt resuscitation (DNAR) should ideally be agreed within the healthcare team, and where appropriate, with the patient or with his or her representative. The overall responsibility rests with the senior clinician, and in some cases this might be a senior nurse. Trusts are required to have a resuscitation policy, and local DNAR arrangements, including the identity of the senior clinician should be clarified within it.

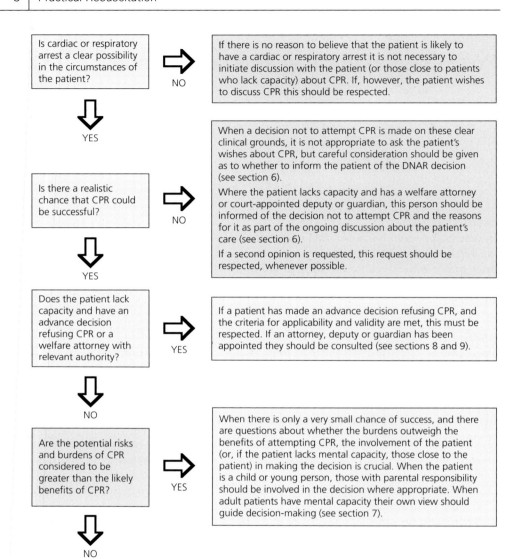

Figure 2.1 Decision-making framework. (Cited in 'Decisions Relating to Cardiopulmonary Resuscitation' (2007; 22). Reproduced with permission of the British Medical Association.)

In general, there is a presumption that unless there is a properly formulated DNAR order, cardiopulmonary resuscitation (CPR) should be initiated. Deliberately ineffective resuscitation attempts, so-called *slow codes*, are considered unethical (Kelly 2007). It is recognised that there may be circumstances where there is no such order in place for a patient for whom resuscitation is clearly not indicated. A junior nurse discovering a collapsed patient in this circumstance would face a difficult decision (Jones 2007). The guidance (Resuscitation Council UK 2007) suggests that a decision not to start CPR in these circumstances should be supported by their senior colleagues and managers. The correctness of the decision turns on the circumstances, and it must be remembered that professional accountability operates here as much as in all over professional decision-making.

In many circumstances, the decision not to attempt CPR is firmly based on the clinical view that it would not be successful, and so should not be offered or attempted. In these cases, it is most likely to be inappropriate to initiate discussion with the patient. In a few cases, patients may request resuscitation even though the team believes that the attempt would be unsuccessful. In this case, there should be sensitive discussion about the likely progress of the disease and the resuscitation attempt. A second opinion may be necessary. The black and white legal position is that clinical staff are under no obligation to provide treatment which they believe is ineffective even if the patient requests it. However, this bald statement of the legal position does not capture the compassion needed to make a decision in these circumstances and communicate it sensitively to the patient whose insistence on resuscitation may reveal inadequate understanding of the prognosis.

In other cases, resuscitation may be successful in that it restores circulation, though this in itself cannot be the sole criterion of a successful resuscitation attempt. The attempt itself is an invasive procedure, and can result in permanent brain damage or other unwanted side effects. The weight given to these side effects can really be assessed only by patients and those who know them. A DNAR decision here weighs the likelihood of benefit and burden, and will include careful consideration of at least the following (Resuscitation Council UK 2007):

- the likely clinical outcome, including the likelihood of successfully restarting the patient's heart and breathing for a sustained period and the level of recovery that can realistically be expected after successful CPR;
- the patient's own ascertainable wishes, including information about previously expressed views, feelings, beliefs and values;
- the patient's human rights, including the right to life and the right to be free of degrading treatment (Wood & Wainright 2007);
- the likelihood of the patient experiencing severe unmanageable pain or suffering;
- the level of awareness the patient has of his or her existence and surroundings.

Patients who decline resuscitation
It is firmly established in law and ethics that a capable patient can refuse any treatment for any reason and any health professional who disregards these wishes is vulnerable to legal challenge. This remains the case where refusal of treatment is

likely to result in the death of the patient where the decision might be considered unwise, even foolhardy by the healthcare team and relatives. Difficulties can arise where there is doubt about whether a patient has the capacity to refuse treatment, and in order to clarify and consolidate existing common law, the Mental Capacity Act (2005) came into force in 2007.

The Mental Capacity Act (2005)

The Mental Capacity Act provides the legal framework for making decisions on behalf of those unable to make them for themselves. Its importance in resuscitation and healthcare, in general, would be difficult to overstate. The Nursing and Midwifery Council's code (2008a; 4) specifically requires that nurses and midwives be aware 'of the legislation regarding mental capacity, ensuring that people who lack capacity remain at the centre of decision making'. The Act largely codifies into statute existing positions established under common law. Readily available and comprehensive guides are available online from the Office of the Public Guardian (2007). The Act affects resuscitation in the following important ways.

Decision-making for patients who lack capacity

It is important to understand that a patient is regarded as incapable only for a specific decision at a specific time. A patient's capacity can be restricted for a number of reasons including dementia, infection and hypoxia. Where patients lack the capacity to make an informed decision, the duty for making a decision in the patient's best interest normally falls not to the family but to the medical team. In some cases, a patient may apparently decline treatment and since the decision to respect the refusal depends hugely on whether the patient is capable of making the decision, there must be a clear process of arriving at a judgement of whether the patient is capable or not. A person is unable to make a decision if he or she has an impairment or a disturbance in the functioning of his or her mind or brain and he or she cannot (Department of Constitutional Affairs 2007; 45):

(1) understand information about the decision to be made;
(2) retain that information in his or her mind;
(3) use or weigh that information as part of the decision-making process; or
(4) communicate his or her decision (by talking, using sign language or any other means).

Advance decisions and lasting power of attorney

The Mental Capacity Act sets out conditions which need to be fulfilled before an advance decision is legally binding. This applies to England and Wales, though the common law of Scotland and Northern Ireland is also likely to support advance decision-making (Resuscitation Council UK 2007). Advance decisions enable patients who have capacity to refuse treatment in the future, when the capacity is lost. They do not have to take a particular form but many charities and voluntary organisations have produced their own versions. But where the decision refuses life-sustaining treatment (including resuscitation), the decision must be in writing, be witnessed, and specifically state that the decision applies even if life is at risk. The person making the advanced decision is responsible for inform-ing the healthcare team of its existence and provisions. It would be wise, though it is not compulsory, for the patients to discuss their wishes with the relatives and their healthcare professionals. Healthcare professionals will be protected from li-ability if they (Department of Constitutional Affairs 2007; 158):

- stop or withhold treatment because they reasonably believe that an advance decision exists, and that it is valid and applicable;
- treat a person because, having taken all practical and appropriate steps to find out if the person has made an advance decision to refuse treatment, they do not know or are not satisfied that a valid and applicable advance decision exists.

Patients can also give another person the authority to make decisions for them when they are unable to make them for themselves. This is known as having lasting power of attorney (LPA). LPAs must be properly documented and reg-istered with the public guardian, and are unable to make decisions relating to life-sustaining treatment unless the document specifically relates to it.

Making and communicating the decision

When a DNAR decision has been made, it is vitally important that it is commu-nicated to all in the healthcare team in the following ways.

- The entry in the medical notes should be clear and unambiguous, with no use of abbreviations.
- The date and the reason for the decision should be clear.
- There should be details of who has been consulted.
- The signature should be easily identifiable.
- A separate entry should also be made in the nursing notes.
- The decision should be reviewed regularly and can be rescinded at any time.

WHEN TO STOP A RESUSCITATION ATTEMPT

The decision-making will depend on a number of factors:

- the environment of the cardiac arrest and access to emergency medical services;
- the interval between cardiac arrest and commencement of basic life support (BLS);
- the interval between BLS and advanced life support (ALS);
- evidence of cardiac death (asystole);
- potential prognosis and co-morbidity (Ambery et al. 2000);
- age of the casualty, but this is a controversial issue (Larkin 2002);
- temperature: hypothermia offers a degree of protection and efforts, prolonged if necessary, should be made to warm the patient (see Chapter 15);
- drug intake prior to cardiac arrest;
- remediable precipitating factors.

Resuscitation should continue if ventricular fibrillation persists and should cease only if asystole is present for more than 20 minutes and in the absence of a re-versible cause (Resuscitation Council UK 2006). It has been recommended that patients should be monitored for 10 minutes after resuscitation efforts have stopped (Maleck *et al.* 1998). The decision should be made by the team leader in consultation with the team.

HAVING FAMILY MEMBERS PRESENT DURING CARDIOPULMONARY RESUSCITATION

The decision whether family members should be permitted to witness the resuscitation of a loved one poses a number of practical, ethical and professional dilemmas for healthcare staff. In recent years, however, the growth of research, public opinion (Mazer *et al.* 2006, Ong *et al.* 2007) and professional expectations have collectively shifted attitudes and eroded some of the perceived barriers.

Critics have been challenged to accept the idea of allowing family members to attend the resuscitation of a loved one on a number of grounds; these include:

- the expansion of the family-centred care movement;
- the growth of the hospice movement;
- public demand for greater openness and transparency;
- the growth of research into family members and healthcare professional perspectives;
- impact of international resuscitation and critical care guidelines supporting the development and implementation of family-friendly policies in this area (Fulbrook *et al.* 2007).

Historically, the pioneering work at the Foote Hospital, Michigan, is credited for promoting worldwide interest in family witnessed resuscitation (FWR; Doyle *et al.* 1987). In this study, relatives who were present reported that their adjustment to the patient's death was made easier by being present; 64% ($n = 30$) believed that their presence was beneficial to the patient and 94% ($n = 44$) indicated that they would attend again.

Excluding family members

Since its introduction, many reasons have been advanced for excluding family members from the resuscitation. Generally, these have been based on cultural factors, speculation and the paternalistic attitudes of healthcare professionals rather than evidence from research (Albarran & Stafford 1999, Baskett & Lim 2004).

The most commonly cited objections include:

- possible family member interference with resuscitation team efforts;
- the immediate and long-term psychological consequences of family presence;
- family member's presence can have an adverse impact on staff performance;
- allowing family members to be present will lead to breaches of patient confidentiality;
- lack of adequate staff resources to supervise and guide family members;
- fears that staff performance will be challenged leading to a rise in medicolegal reprisals.

Arguments for FWR

Because of conflicting attitudes, the practice of allowing family members to observe the resuscitation of a loved one has been slow to evolve. However, while families who unexpectedly are faced with a situation involving the resuscitation and possible death of a loved one entrust the care of the patient to healthcare professionals they nevertheless wish to be present because of:

- a sense of duty and obligation;
- a desire to remain connected with the patient;
- a need to understand and be reassured about their loved one's health and that they are being cared for (Eichhorn *et al.* 2001, Weslien *et al.* 2006).

Being present has been reported to be beneficial to family members by enabling them to:

- observe that the resuscitation team did everything that could be done;
- reduce any misconceptions and misunderstandings of life-saving procedures;
- understand the severity of a loved one's condition and prognosis;
- remain emotionally connected to the patient and a life of shared memories;
- provide comfort and support to their loved ones;
- advise team about the patient's interests and participate in decisions affecting their loved ones;
- feel that, in the case of an unsuccessful resuscitation, they shared the last moments with their loved ones, accept the death and begin the process of closure and grief;
- suffer reduced grief and achieve earlier psychological adjustment (Duran *et al.* 2007, Eichhorn *et al.* 2001, Holzhauser *et al.* 2006, Meyers *et al.* 2000, Robinson *et al.* 1998).

Additionally, family members who attend the resuscitation of a loved one stay focused on the patient, recognise when it is inappropriate to remain at the bedside and are unrepentant over their decisions to be present (Holzhauser *et al.* 2006, Robinson *et al.* 1998). Patients and families also appear to recognise that their presence must be balanced with enabling the resuscitation team to perform their duties uninterrupted and healthcare staff should be allowed to make discretionary judgements in the interest of patients and relatives (Albarran *et al.* 2007, Weslien *et al.* 2006). Breaches of confidentiality are less of a concern for patients; indeed, many accept that this may be necessary in facilitating family members to make decisions about further treatment options (Albarran *et al.* 2007).

Patient perceptions of personal benefit

Experiences of patients who have undergone resuscitation and survived or underwent invasive procedures are scarce. Patients generally agree that relatives should always be given the option to be present and it is important because families are able to:

- reduce a patient's feelings of isolation, insecurity and fear;
- provide emotional comfort beyond the scope of healthcare professionals;
- maintain family bonds;
- humanise the environment enabling the patient to be viewed in a social context (Albarran *et al.* 2007, Eichhorn *et al.* 2001).

While some patients may not wish to have families present during their resuscitation, those with a positive disposition may sanction this but only under certain conditions. Therefore, it is important, where feasible, to assess their views and preferences of patients, record and communicate these with the clinical team. This information should enable healthcare staff to be aware of how to manage the patients' interests in such eventualities.

Supporting the family member during resuscitation of a relative

In managing such emotionally charged situations, a hospital-wide policy is vital for directing the practice of healthcare staff; however, a few have these in place (Fulbrook *et al.* 2005). A recent European position statement provides a series of statements to support the delivery of care (see Box 2.1; Fulbrook *et al.* 2007). The position statement is underpinned by the premise that family members are critical to improving the health, recovery and well-being of patients.

Ensuring that a family's experience of being present is positive, despite the exceptional circumstances, demands detailed planning involving members of the multi-disciplinary team (Baskett *et al.* 2005). A family member's decision not to witness the resuscitation of a loved one should be respected and individuals should not feel guilty or coerced into changing their mind. Extending an invitation to a family to be present during the resuscitation of a loved one needs to be conveyed in neutral and non-judgemental terms.

Box 2.1   Joint position statement on the presence of family members during cardiopulmonary resuscitation.

Position statement

1. All patients have the right to have a family member present during resuscitation.
2. The patient's family members should be offered the opportunity to be present during the resuscitation of a relative.
3. Support should be provided by an appropriately qualified healthcare professional whose responsibility is to care for family members witnessing cardiopulmonary resuscitation.
4. Professional counselling should be offered to family members who have witnessed a resuscitation event.
5. All members of the resuscitation team who were involved in a resuscitation attempt when family members were present should participate in team debriefing.
6. Family presence during resuscitation should be incorporated into the curricula of cardiopulmonary resuscitation training programmes.
7. All wards and critical care units should have multi-disciplinary written guidelines on the presence of family members during cardiopulmonary resuscitation.

Fulbrook *et al.* 2007; Reprinted with permission of Connect Healthcare Publishing Ltd and EfCCNa.

- The resuscitation needs to be performed competently and by a clear team leader, within an environment that is welcoming and supportive of family members.
- Family members need to be clear that their decision to be present is a voluntary one.
- Relatives need to be briefed and advised what to expect prior to entering the resuscitation room.
- Regular explanations should be provided in simple terms and avoiding jargon. Confirming understanding is vital to ensure visitors comprehend the sequence of events and to help reduce any misunderstandings.
- Family members need to be aware that they may observe procedures, including those of an invasive nature, and which the patient may respond by displaying involuntary actions (e.g. convulsions post-defibrillation).
- There may be occasions that family members may be asked to step away from resuscitation for safety reasons or to maintain the patient's dignity.
- Preparing family members to be present must also entail altering them that should resuscitation attempts fail, treatment may need to be abandoned. However, any decision made to withdraw care can be taken only by a senior physician. The views of family members may be sought, but the decision to stop resuscitation will not rest with them (Department of Constitutional Affairs, 2007).
- Provision should be made to allow family members to ask questions and have any issues clarified. Some family members may wish to view the deceased for a final time, as many of them find this helpful (Haas, 2003). Offering honest, compassionate, individualised information and support can positively influence the bereavement experience for family members (Li *et al.* 2002). Advice about registering the death and support services available should also be provided.

ROLE OF THE HEALTHCARE PROFESSIONAL AT RESUSCITATION

The initial management sequence

A respiratory or cardiac arrest may occur at any time and at any place within the healthcare environment. Though these may be unproblematic, complications can exist, such as the patient who is:

- in a wheelchair with a bilateral amputation of his or her legs;
- prone on the operating table mid procedure;
- collapsed whilst on the toilet and has become wedged between the toilet and the cubicle wall;
- in the bath;
- on the treadmill during an exercise test in the cardiology department;
- found hanging from the fire escape following a suicide attempt.

It may be a member of the staff who has been arrested in the hospital canteen or car park. In responding to any situation, it is imperative that first responders ensure their own safety. Only then can first responders begin to deal with the situation, the following issues need to be considered.

Call for appropriate help and assess casualty

If the casualty fails to respond to verbal commands or to gentle shaking, perform an assessment for signs of life and if these are absent, shout for help (see Chapter 6). If other members of the team are present, get someone to call the cardiac arrest number and fetch the emergency equipment. All staff should also be aware of where the nearest cardiac arrest trolley and defibrillator are located.

The casualty should be rapidly placed unto a supine position to enable access to the airway and pulse. Do not delay in checking for a pulse, but start to give 30 chest compressions followed by two ventilations and continue until assistance is available. For a detailed discussion on subsequent actions, refer to Chapter 6. If the patient is in bed, it is not absolutely essential for the headboard to be removed before airway management begins. Ensure that the mattress type is suitable for performing resuscitation. There are some mattresses that are unsuitable when chest compressions are being performed on a patient, such as an air mattress that will need to be deflated in an appropriate manner.

The cardiac arrest team members and how to work with them

Most cardiac arrest teams will consist of the following healthcare workers:

- medical senior house officer (SHO) and/or registrar (generally assume team leader role);
- medical house officer (HO);
- anaesthetist (and often an assistant such as an operating department practitioner/assistant (ODP/ODA) or intensive care/anaesthetic nurse);
- senior nurse (may be departmental senior nurse or clinical site manager);
- resuscitation officer (RO).

In addition to the team, there are likely to be several staff members from the ward or department who will stay with the patient and work with the team. These members are important, as often they will have the best knowledge of the patient.

To ensure a coordinated approach, the Resuscitation Council UK (2000) suggests that the cardiac arrest team meets daily, preferably at the beginning of any new shift, and appoints a team leader in the event of a cardiac arrest call.

The following healthcare professionals perform essential skills.

- *Medical registrar* – acting as cardiac arrest team leader, standing back from the patient to achieve a good overview of the activities of the team and give clear directions accordingly.
- *Medical house officer* – attempting to achieve intravenous access so that drugs can be administered quickly.
- *Anaesthetist* – managing the airway with bag-valve-mask ventilation.
- *Intensive care nurse* – assisting the anaesthetist.
- *Student nurse* – performing chest compressions under the supervision and support of the intensive care nurse.
- *Ward sister* – performing defibrillation.

The Resuscitation Council UK (2003) gives very clear guidance on the role of the cardiac arrest team leader and the individual team members.

POST-ARREST

Following any resuscitation attempt, successful or not, a number of tasks will need to be undertaken. These are considered in more detail in Chapter 14 and will include:

- completion of the cardiac arrest audit or report form;
- restocking the cardiac arrest trolley;
- dealing with relatives;
- debriefing for the cardiac arrest team.

Professional accountability for maintaining skills and competence and off-duty issues

While you may not have to resuscitate anyone throughout your professional career, the Nursing and Midwifery Council (2008a; 7) nevertheless advises that nurses, "must have the knowledge and skills for safe and effective practice when working without direct supervision". Nurses "must recognise and work within the limits of their competence". Individuals must "keep their knowledge and skills up to date throughout their working life". Nurses must take part in appropriate learning and practice activities that maintain and develop their competence and performance. Because competence and skills decay, if not used, the need for regular updating to achieve a satisfactory standard of performance during resuscitation remains the responsibility of individual professionals.

In most situations, there is a clear moral duty for healthcare staff to attend a casualty when not at work but at present there is no legal requirement to do so in the UK. Unlike its previous version, the Nursing and Midwifery Council code (NMC 2008a; 7) does not explicitly state that nurses have a professional duty to offer care to a casualty. However, other NMC guidance does make it clear that the professional duty to care continues even when nurses are not at work (NMC 2008b), and so an individual failing to offer assistance may be called to account by the Nursing and Midwifery Council. There is some concern that legal action may be brought as a result of a resuscitation attempt in the community (Resuscitation Council UK 2000). The paucity of cases in this area makes it difficult to come to any definite conclusions but healthcare professionals are advised:

- to follow guidelines recommended by authoritative bodies;
- to check the extent of personal indemnity insurance.

A discussion paper with further advice is available from the Resuscitation Council UK (2000).

REVIEW OF LEARNING

- ❏ Resuscitation is not always appropriate in persons who suffer from cardiac arrest.
- ❏ Patients' wishes on their resuscitation status should usually be sought and respected.
- ❏ Family members should be allowed to witness resuscitation attempts provided certain conditions are met.

❏ There is a professional duty for healthcare professionals to offer emergency treatment.
❏ Good assessment and consideration of the environment are essential in the initial management of the arrested patient.
❏ Resuscitation may be attempted prior to the arrival of the team, and then continue with effective team working.
❏ Following resuscitation, a number of tasks need to be completed such as debriefing and audit form completion

CONCLUSION

In recent years, a number of developments and policies designed to guide practitioners have emerged. These have related to DNAR, living wills, mental capacity and incapacity and FWR, all of which impact on decisions relating to cardiopulmonary resuscitation. This chapter considers a wide range of important professional, ethical and legal issues associated with resuscitation events. The remaining chapters support the development of clinical competence through presenting a comprehensive evidence base in resuscitation: recognition and response.

REFERENCES

Albarran, J.W., Moule, P., Benger, J., McMahon-Parkes, K. & Lockyer L. (2007) *Witnessed Resuscitation: What Do Patients Really Want?* University of the West of England, Bristol.

Albarran, J.W. & Stafford, H. (1999) Resuscitation and family presence: implications for nurses in critical areas. *Advancing Clinical Nursing* **3** (1), 11–19.

Ambery, P., King, B. & Banerjee, M. (2000) Does concurrent or previous illness accurately predict cardiac arrest survival? *Resuscitation* **47**, 267–71.

American Heart Association/International Liaison Committee on Resuscitation (2000) Guidelines for cardiopulmonary resuscitation and emergency cardiovascular care. *Circulation* **102** (suppl 8), 1–374.

Baskett, P.J.F. & Lim, A. (2004) The varying ethical attitudes towards family witnessed resuscitation. *Resuscitation* **64**, 263–7.

Baskett, P.J.F., Steen, P.A. & Bossaert, L. (2005) European Council guidelines for resuscitation 2005. Section 8: the ethics of resuscitation and end of life decisions. *Resuscitation* **67** (suppl 1), S171–80.

Department of Constitutional Affairs (2007) *Mental Capacity Act Code of Practice*. TSO, London. Available online at: http://www.justice.gov.uk/docs/mca-cp.pdf.

Doyle, C.J., Post, H., Maino, J., Keefe, M. & Rhee, K. (1987) Family participation during resuscitation: an option. *Annals of Emergency Medicine* **16** (6), 673–5.

Duran, C., Oman, K., Jordan, J., Koziel, V. & Szymanski, D. (2007) Attitudes and beliefs about family presence: a survey of healthcare providers, patients' families and patients. *American Journal of Critical Care* **16** (3), 270–79.

Eichhorn, D., Meyers, T., Guzzetta, C.E., Clark, A. & Klein, J. (2001) Family presence during invasive procedures and resuscitation: hearing the voice of the patient. *American Journal of Nursing* **101** (5), 48–55.

Fulbrook, P., Albarran, J.W. & Latour, J. (2005) A European survey of critical care nurses' attitudes and experiences of having family members' present during cardiopulmonary resuscitation. *International Journal of Nursing Studies* **42**, 557–68.

Fulbrook, P., Latour, J., Albarran, J.W. *et al.* (2007) The presence of family members during cardiopulmonary resuscitation: European Federation of Critical Care Nursing Associations, European and Neonatal Intensive Care and European Society of Cardiology Council on

Cardiovascular Nursing and Allied Professions Joint position statement. *CONNECT: The World of Critical Care Nursing* **5** (4), 86–8.

Haas, F. (2003) Bereavement care: seeing the body. *Nursing Standard* **17** (28), 33–7.

Holzhauser, K., Finucane, J. & De Vries, S.M. (2006) Family presence during resuscitation: a randomised controlled trial of the impact of family presence. *Australasian Emergency Nursing Journal* **8**, 139–47.

Jones, J. (2007) Do not resuscitate: reflections on an ethical dilemma. *Nursing Standard* **21** (46), 35–9.

Kelly, J. (2007) Literature review: decision-making regarding slow resuscitation. *Journal of Clinical Nursing* **16**, 1989–96.

Larkin, G.L. (2002) Termination of resuscitation: the art of clinical decision making. *Current Opinion in Critical Care* **8** (3), 224–9.

Li, S.P., Chan C. & Lee, D. (2002) Helpfulness of nursing actions to suddenly bereaved family members in an accident and emergency setting in Hong Kong. *Journal of Advanced Nursing* **40** (2), 170–80.

Maleck, W.H., Piper, S.N., Triem, J., Boldt, J. & Zittel, F.U. (1998) Unexpected return of spontaneous circulation after cessation of resuscitation (Lazarus phenomenon). *Resuscitation* **39**, 125–8.

Mazer, M.A., Cox, L.A. & Capon, J.A. (2006) The public's attitude and perception concerning witnessed resuscitation. *Critical Care Medicine* **34** (2), 2925–8.

Meyers, T., Eichhorn, D., Guzetta, C.E. *et al.* (2000) Family presence during invasive procedures and resuscitation: the experience of family members, nurses and physicians. *American Journal of Nursing* **100** (2), 32–42.

Nursing and Midwifery Council (2008a) *The Code. Standards of Conduct, Performance and Ethics for Nurses and Midwives*. Nursing and Midwifery Council, London.

Nursing and Midwifery Council (2008b). *Duty of Care (A–Z Advice Sheets)*. Nursing and Midwifery Council, London.

Office of the Public Guardian (2007) *Making Decisions: A Guide for People Working in Health and Social Care*. Available online at: http://www.publicguardian.gov.uk/docs/making-decisions-opg603-1207.pdf.

Ong, M., Chung, W. & Mei, S. (2007) Comparing attitudes of the public and medical staff towards witnessed resuscitation in an Asian population. *Resuscitation* **73**, 103–8.

Resuscitation Council UK (2000) *The Legal Status of Those Who Attempt Resuscitation*. Resuscitation Council UK, London. Available online at: www.resus.org.uk/pages/legal.htm.

Resuscitation Council UK (2003*) Advanced Life Support Course Provider Manual Appendix: The Cardiac Arrest Team Leader and Team*, 4th edn. Resuscitation Council UK, London.

Resuscitation Council UK (2006) *Advanced Life Support*, 5th edn. Resuscitation Council UK, London.

Resuscitation Council UK (2007) *Decisions Relating to Cardiopulmonary Resuscitation*. A joint statement from the Royal College of Nursing the Resuscitation Council UK and British Medical Association. Available online at: http://www.resus.org.uk/pages/dnar.pdf.

Robinson, S.M., Mackenzie-Ross, S., Campbell Hewson, G.L., Egleston, C.V. & Prevost, A.T. (1998) Psychological effect of witnessed resuscitation on bereaved relatives. *Lancet* **352** (9128), 614–17.

Wagner, J.M. (2004) Lived experience of critically ill patients' family members during cardiopulmonary resuscitation. *American Journal of Critical Care* **13**, 416–20.

Weslien, M., Nilstun, T., Lundqvist, A. & Fridlund, B. (2006) Narratives about resuscitation – family members differ about presence. *European Journal of Cardiovascular Nursing* **5**, 68–74.

Wood, J. & Wainright, P. (2007) cardiopulmonary resuscitation: nurses and the law. *Nursing Standard* **22** (4), 35–40.

Section 2

Prevention and Preparation

3 | Recognising the Critically Ill Patient and Preventing Cardiorespiratory Arrest

Jackie Younker

INTRODUCTION

The survival rates following cardiac arrest are poor. In approximately 80% of cases, there is deterioration in clinical signs during the few hours before the cardiac arrest. Early recognition of the critically ill patient and appropriate immediate response will hopefully prevent some cardiac arrests, deaths and admissions to intensive care units. Track and trigger systems are useful in identifying changes in vital signs and alerting staff to a deterioration in a patient's condition. This may prompt staff to call an identified medical emergency team (MET) or critical care outreach team or the most appropriate expert help. The use of the ABCDE approach provides a systematic tool for assessing and treating all critically ill patients and should be used for all patients.

AIMS

This chapter discusses how to use a systematic ABCDE approach to recognise and respond to the critically ill patient.

LEARNING OUTCOMES

At the end of the chapter, the reader will be able to:

❏ understand the importance of early recognition of the critically ill patient;
❏ recognise causes of cardiorespiratory arrest in adults;
❏ describe how the critically ill patient should be *identified* and *treated using the ABCDE approach*;
❏ identify the importance of *calling for expert help rapidly*.

THE CRITICALLY ILL PATIENT

Most people who have a cardiac arrest die. Those who do survive an in-hospital cardiac arrest most likely have a witnessed and monitored ventricular fibrillation (VF) arrest and receive a prompt and successful defibrillation.

Cardiorespiratory arrest in a hospital is not usually sudden or unpredictable. Often there is a gradual deterioration in clinical signs during the few hours before the cardiac arrest. These patients often have slow, progressive physiological deterioration that may go unnoticed or if recognised is ineffectively managed (NCEPOD 2005). Common problems are hypotension and hypoxia (Kause *et al.*

2004). Patients in this group usually have a non-shockable rhythm (PEA or asystole – see Chapters 7 and 10) and the survival rate to hospital discharge is very low, i.e. fewer than 20% of adult patients (Peberdy *et al.* 2003).

Some cardiac arrests, deaths and admissions to intensive care units may be prevented by early recognition and effective treatment of critically ill patients (Nolan *et al.* 2005). Cardiorespiratory resuscitation may not be appropriate for some and for those who choose not to be resuscitated. Early recognition will help to identify them and facilitate a do not attempt resuscitation (DNAR, see Chapter 2) status for the patient (Nolan *et al.* 2005).

Recognising critical illness

The clinical signs of critical illness tend to look the same whatever the underlying process because they reflect failing respiratory, cardiovascular and neurologic systems. This will be discussed later in detail. Physiological deterioration is common on general wards; however, measurement and recording of physiological observations (e.g. heart rate, blood pressure, respiratory rate and temperature) is often inconsistent and less frequent than desired (Harrison *et al.* 2005). Simply improving measurement and recording of vital signs, particularly respiratory rate, may help to predict patients at risk for cardiorespiratory arrest.

Many hospitals in the UK and other countries use track and trigger systems (e.g. early warning systems and calling criteria) to help detect critical illness early. There are a variety of systems in use throughout the UK, but the principle is the same. Points are allocated to measurements of routine vital signs. Any deviations from the 'normal' range will prompt the next level of intervention such as increasing the frequency of observations, calling the doctor or activating a resuscitation or MET. Figure 3.1 provides an example of calling criteria. No particular track and trigger or early warning system has been proven to be better than the others (Smith *et al.* 2008). The National Institute for Clinical Excellence (NICE 2007) in the UK has provided guidelines for all wards to have a track and trigger system in place appropriate to local needs.

Responding to critical illness

Recognising the critically ill patient and calling for help early will help to prevent cardiorespiratory arrest. There are different approaches to providing help depending on the hospital.

- MET – in some hospitals, the traditional 'cardiac arrest' team has been replaced by the MET to respond to patients who have deteriorated as well as those who have arrested. The MET usually includes medical and nursing staff from acute care areas with training and expertise to treat the critically ill patient, usually with simple measures such as oxygen and intravenous (IV) fluids. Early involvement may reduce cardiac arrests, deaths and unanticipated intensive care admissions. The benefits of the MET have not been proved (Nolan *et al.* 2005).
- Critical care outreach – this has been developed in some hospitals in the UK as a way of treating critically ill patients on the ward. Outreach services vary from hospital to hospital with some providing nursing coverage by individual nurses and others using a team to cover 24 hours per day, seven days per week.

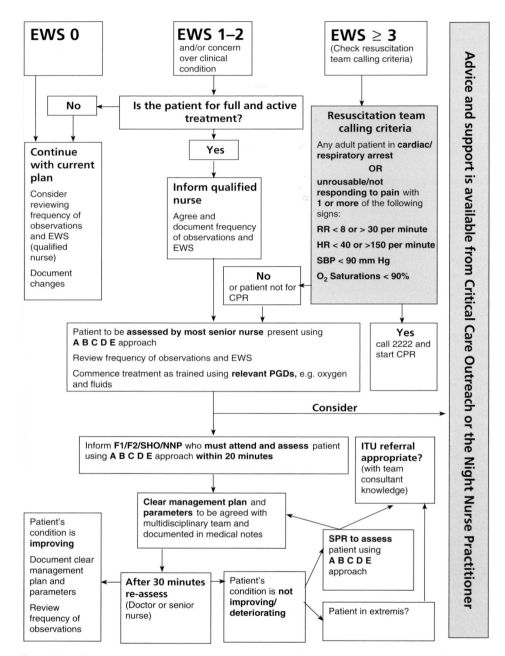

Figure 3.1 Early warning score system. (Reproduced with permission of Gloucestershire Hospitals NHS Foundation Trust.)

The goal is to reduce ward deaths, postoperative adverse events, admissions and re-admissions to intensive care units and increase survival. There is limited evidence to prove their benefits (McGaughey *et al*. 2007).

All patients should be monitored using a track and trigger system to detect physiological changes and response teams should be provided based on local needs and resources. The key is immediate response for all patients at high risk of cardiorespiratory arrest (NICE 2007).

Causes of cardiorespiratory arrest

Cardiorespiratory arrest is most likely caused by a primary airway, breathing or cardiovascular problem (Resuscitation Council UK 2006).

Airway

The airway can become obstructed for many reasons including:

- blood;
- vomit;
- a foreign body;
- epiglottitis;
- pharyngeal swelling (e.g. oedema and infection);
- bronchial secretions;
- central nervous system depression;
- bronchospasm;
- laryngospasm.

Recognising airway problems

In complete airway obstruction, there are no breath sounds. If the patient attempts to breathe, there will be a seesaw (paradoxical) breathing pattern, where the abdomen moves in as the chest wall moves out during attempted inspiration. In the unconscious patient, obstruction of the pharynx by the tongue is the most common cause of complete airway obstruction. This is commonly, but inaccurately, known as 'swallowing the tongue' and occurs as muscle tone is lost. If the airway is not opened and cleared quickly by the use of the simple techniques described in Chapter 9, expert help must be called immediately.

Breathing is often noisy in partial airway obstruction. A conscious patient may be able to indicate that there is something wrong and there is often considerable distress. Treatment is directed at the cause and may involve simple airway opening manoeuvres with adjuncts and patient positioning, such as the recovery position. If there is no improvement or if advanced techniques, for example tracheal intubation, are required, senior help should be called without delay (see Chapter 9).

Breathing problem

Breathing problems may be acute or chronic and be continuous or intermittent. A breathing problem that is severe enough to cause apnoea will rapidly lead to a cardiac arrest. Respiratory arrest usually occurs due to a combination of factors (Resuscitation Council UK 2006). For example, a patient with chronic respiratory disease may have symptoms exacerbated by a chest infection or muscle weakness. This can lead to exhaustion and further depress respiratory function. Failure to breathe adequately will lead to insufficient oxygenation of the blood and cardiac arrest will eventually occur.

Breathing inadequacy can be classified into problems with respiratory drive, respiratory effort and lung disorders.

- Respiratory drive – respiratory drive is regulated by the central nervous system. Central nervous system depression may be caused by head injury, intracerebral disease, hypercarbia, certain metabolic disorders (e.g. diabetes mellitus) and drugs. Central nervous system depression may decrease or abolish the patient's drive to breathe (Guyton and Hall 2005).
- Respiratory effort – the diaphragm and intercostal muscles are the main muscles used in breathing. The diaphragm is innervated at the level of the third, fourth and fifth segments of the spinal cord. Severe cervical cord damage above this level will make spontaneous breathing impossible. The intercostal muscles are innervated at the level of their respective ribs and may be paralysed by a spinal cord lesion above this level. Breathing may be impaired by restrictive chest abnormalities (kyphoscoliosis) or pain from fractured ribs or sternum. Other diseases may lead to muscle weakness or nerve damage (e.g. Guillain–Barre syndrome, multiple sclerosis). Generalised weakness of respiratory muscles may also occur with chronic malnutrition and severe long-term illness (Guyton and Hall 2005).
- Lung disorders – severe lung disease will impair gas exchange. Infection, aspiration, exacerbation of chronic obstructive pulmonary disease, asthma, pulmonary embolus, lung contusion, acute respiratory distress syndrome (ARDS) and pulmonary oedema are common causes (Resuscitation Council UK 2006). Lung function is also impaired by a pneumothorax or haemothorax.

Recognising breathing problems

A conscious patient will look distressed and complain of feeling short of breath. A simple and useful indicator of breathing problems is a fast respiratory rate (>30 breaths/min) (Smith *et al.* 2002). Signs of hypoxia and hypercarbia include irritability, confusion, lethargy and a decrease in the level of consciousness. The patient may have cyanosis, but this is a late sign. Pulse oximetry is non-invasive and a useful way to measure the adequacy of oxygenation. An arterial blood gas will be helpful in measuring the adequacy of ventilation and provides values for partial carbon dioxide tension ($PaCO_2$) and pH. A patient with late signs of severe respiratory problems will have a decreased pH and an increased $PaCO_2$. All patients with breathing problems and hypoxia should have oxygen as soon as possible (Resuscitation Council UK 2006). Further support with ventilation may be necessary (see Chapter 9 for a detailed review).

Cardiovascular problem

Cardiovascular problems may be caused by primary heart disease or heart abnormalities secondary to other problems.

- Primary heart problems – the most common reason for cardiac arrest is an arrhythmia caused by ischaemia or myocardial infarction. Box 3.1 provides a list

---

Box 3.1   Causes of ventricular fibrillation.

- Acute coronary syndromes
- Hypertensive heart disease
- Heart valve disease
- Hereditary heart diseases
- Acidosis
- Abnormal electrolyte levels (e.g. potassium, magnesium and calcium)
- Drugs (e.g. antiarrhythmic drugs, tricyclic antidepressants and digoxin)
- Electrocution
- Hypothermia

Adapted from Resuscitation Council UK 2006.

---

of causes of VF. Sudden cardiac arrest may also occur with cardiac failure, cardiac tamponade, cardiac rupture, myocarditis and hypertrophic cardiomyopathy.

- Secondary heart problems – changes elsewhere in the body will affect the heart. A primary respiratory arrest (e.g. apnoea, airway obstruction, asphyxia and tension pneumothorax) will result in a secondary cardiac arrest due to decreased oxygenation of the heart.
- Acute coronary syndromes (ACS) – these comprise unstable angina, non-ST elevation myocardial infarction (NSTEMI) and ST elevation myocardial infarction (STEMI). These syndromes arise from the same pathophysiology; thrombosis of a coronary artery is triggered by rupture or fissuring or an atheromatous plaque in the coronary artery. Myocardial blood flow is reduced and the extent of this determines the syndrome (Jowett and Thompson 2003).

Recognising cardiovascular problems

General signs and symptoms of heart disease include chest pain, shortness of breath, tachycardia, bradycardia, high respiratory rate, hypotension, poor peripheral perfusion, change in level of consciousness, syncope and decreased urinary output. Acute myocardial infarction (AMI) usually presents with:

- pain, which is the initial response to myocardial ischaemia. Typically, the pain is central and gripping in nature. Commonly, it radiates to the left arm, though pain can be reported anywhere in the chest, arms, neck, jaw and teeth (Albarran and Tagney 2007);
- nausea and vomiting;
- hypotension;
- anxiety;
- tachycardia;
- pale, clammy skin.

A history of sustained acute chest pain with acute ST segment elevation on the 12-lead ECG is the basis for a diagnosis of STEMI.

Some patients present with chest pain suggestive of AMI, but have less specific ECG changes such as ST segment depression or T wave inversion. If laboratory tests show release of Troponin, this indicates that myocardial damage has occurred. This is an NSTEMI.

Patients who have an unprovoked, prolonged episode of chest pain without definite ECG or laboratory evidence of AMI are considered to be having unstable angina.

Treatment for an ACS should be immediate and includes (Arntz *et al.* 2005):

M – morphine (or diamorphine). This should be given intravenously. Cannulation is a priority;
O – oxygen, in a high concentration;
N – nitroglycerine (GTN) spray, to dilate the coronary arteries;
A – aspirin 300 mg orally – crushed or chewed.

Further treatment will depend on the extent of the acute coronary treatment and may include thrombolytic therapy or percutaneous coronary intervention.

Secondary cardiac arrests may be prevented by treating the underlying cause. For example, optimising vital organ perfusion using early goal-directed therapy decreases the risk of death in severe sepsis (Dellinger *et al.* 2008). Other interventions may include correcting underlying electrolyte or acid–base disturbances, and treatment to normalise heart rate, rhythm and output. Some interventions will require expert help, but should be considered (e.g. fluid therapy to manipulate cardiac filling and vasoactive drug administration).

The ABCDE approach to assessment
A systematic approach to assessing and treating all critically ill patients will help in prevention of cardiorespiratory arrest (Smith *et al.* 2002). The **A**irway, **B**reathing, **C**irculation, **D**isability and **E**xposure (ABCDE) approach should be used to assess and guide treatment of critically ill patients. It is important to do a complete initial assessment and re-assess responses to treatment regularly. Any life-threatening problems must be treated before moving on to the next part of the assessment. Key points include calling for help early, using all members of the team to undertake simultaneous tasks and communicating effectively. This approach can be used regardless of your level of training and experience in clinical assessment or treatment. Your level of clinical knowledge and skill will determine the detail of your assessment and level of intervention. Recognising and responding to problems early will hopefully keep the patient alive and achieve some clinical improvement.

There are a few basic steps to take with all patients. First, ensure your personal safety and look at the patient in general to see if the patient looks unwell. Asking simple questions such as 'how are you?' or if the patient appears unconscious, shake him gently and ask, 'are you all right?' If the patient responds normally, you will know the airway is open, the patient is breathing and there is adequate brain perfusion. Speaking in short sentences may indicate breathing problems. If the patient fails to respond, this is a clear sign of critical illness. Basic monitoring should be initiated promptly including pulse, blood pressure and respiration rate. A pulse oximeter and ECG monitor should be applied as soon as possible for all critically ill patients. Insertion of an IV cannula should also be done as quickly as possible with blood being sent for further investigations.

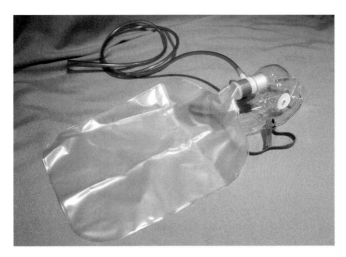

Figure 3.2 A non-rebreathing mask.

A – Airway

Assess the airway first. Any airway obstruction is an emergency and it is important to get expert help immediately. Signs of airway obstruction include:

- paradoxical chest and abdominal movements (seesaw respirations) and the use of accessory muscles of respiration;
- central cyanosis (e.g. blue lips and mouth) – be aware of, this is a late sign;
- partial obstruction may present with noisy breathing; complete obstruction presents with no breath sounds at the nose or mouth.

Simple methods of airway clearance may be all that are needed. These include airway opening manoeuvres, suction and insertion of a nasopharyngeal or oropharyngeal airway. Tracheal intubation may be needed if other techniques fail (see Chapter 9).

Oxygen should be given at a high concentration using a mask with an oxygen reservoir (non-rebreathing mask; see Figure 3.2). A mask with a reservoir bag can deliver an inspired oxygen concentration of approximately 85% at flows of 10–15 L/min. Oxygen may be given with a self-inflating bag if the patient's trachea is intubated. The aim is to achieve a normal oxygen saturation of 97–100%. A pulse oximeter may be used to guide oxygen delivery. This may not always be realistic in the sickest patients and it may be possible to only achieve oxygen saturations of 90–92%. Arterial blood gas monitoring should also be used to guide oxygen therapy (Nolan *et al*. 2005).

B – Breathing

Life-threatening conditions may be impairing breathing (e.g. acute severe asthma, pulmonary oedema, tension pneumothorax or massive haemothorax). These should be diagnosed and treated immediately. Breathing is assessed using the look, listen and feel approach. General signs of respiratory distress include sweating, central cyanosis, use of the accessory muscles of respiration and abdominal breathing. Other important points for assessing breathing include:

- Count the respiratory rate. A normal rate is 12–20 breaths/min. It is useful to compare readings with previously recorded measurements. A high or increasing respiratory rate is a marker of critical illness and a warning that sudden deterioration may occur (Peberdy *et al.* 2003).
- Assess the chest during breathing, noting the depth of each breath, the pattern of respiration and whether chest expansion is normal and equal on both sides. Any chest deformities may increase the risk of deterioration in the ability to breathe normally.
- Measure the oxygen saturation using pulse oximetry and record this along with the inspired oxygen concentration. A patient receiving oxygen does not necessarily have adequate ventilation. It is possible that the patient is breathing inadequately and has a high partial pressure of carbon dioxide ($PaCO_2$).
- Listen for audible breathing noises such as stridor or wheezing that suggest partial airway obstruction. Rattling airway noises may indicate secretions in the airway, usually related to the patient's inability to cough or breathe deeply.
- Chest percussion and auscultation may also provide useful assessment information. Perform these if you are trained to do so.
- All critically ill patients should receive high flow oxygen. If the patient's depth or rate of breathing is inadequate or if the patient has stopped breathing, use a pocket mask or two-person bag-mask ventilation while calling for expert urgent help (see Chapter 9).

C – Circulation

A failure to perfuse vital organs can lead to permanent damage and death. A rapid assessment of the circulation is therefore vital. In almost all medical and surgical emergencies, hypovolaemia should be considered as the likeliest cause of shock. Any patient with cool peripheries and a high heart rate should receive IV fluid unless there is an obvious contraindication (e.g. chest pain and cardiac failure) (Nolan *et al.* 2005). Circulation assessment includes:

- Observation of the hands and fingers for colour and temperature. Blue, mottled, cool hands indicate decreased blood perfusion to the peripheries.
- Measurement of capillary refill time – normal refill time is <2 seconds. A prolonged time suggests poor peripheral perfusion, but this can be affected by other factors such as cold surroundings, poor lighting or old age.
- Pulse measurement – a normal rate is considered 60 and 100 beats/min, though as this varies between individuals, changes in the recorded trend rather than one-off values are important. A thin thready pulse with cool peripheries can indicate low cardiac output, e.g. hypovolaemia. A full, bounding pulse with warm peripheries can indicate sepsis. An irregular pulse can indicate cardiac rhythm abnormalities.
- Blood pressure measurement – it remains an important measure of critical illness, though a reduction in blood pressure from baseline values is often a

delayed sign of shock, as heart rate and force of contraction and peripheral vasoconstriction act to normalise blood pressure. A low diastolic blood pressure suggests arterial vasodilation (e.g. anaphylaxis or sepsis).

- Looking for obvious signs of bleeding from wounds or drains. A patient may be bleeding in the body cavity without evidence of blood in surgical drains, so it is also important to consider concealed bleeding.

Treatment of cardiovascular collapse is aimed at fluid replacement, control of bleeding and restoring tissue perfusion. Conditions that are immediately life-threatening (e.g. cardiac tamponade, haemorrhage or septic shock) must be identified and treated urgently. Intravenous cannulation should be established with a large bore cannulae as soon as possible. Blood may be taken during cannulation and sent for routine haematological, biochemical, coagulation and microbiological investigations. A rapid fluid challenge should be given of 500 mL of warmed crystalloid solution (e.g. Hartmann's or 0.9% saline) over 5–10 minutes if the patient has a normal blood pressure. Hypotensive patients should receive 1 L of warmed crystalloid solution (e.g. Hartmann's or 0.9% saline). If the patient has known cardiac failure, give 250 mL of fluid and monitor the patient closely (Resuscitation Council UK 2006). Pulse and blood pressure monitoring should continue regularly (5 minutes), aiming for the patient's normal blood pressure or a systolic blood pressure of >100 mm Hg. The fluid challenge may be repeated if the patient does not improve.

Any patient with primary chest pain and a suspected ACS should be assessed using the ABCDE approach – using the treatment of oxygen, morphine, nitroglycerine and aspirin mentioned above as well as obtaining a 12-lead ECG.

D – Disability

Many acutely ill patients have changes in their conscious level. Common reasons include profound hypoxia, hypercapnia, cerebral hypoperfusion due to hypotension or the recent administration of analgesics or sedative drugs. Reviewing and treating the ABCs will prove useful in excluding hypoxia and hypotension. The patient's drug chart will provide information about recent drugs given. If available, the appropriate antagonist agent should be given (e.g. naloxone for opioid overdose) (Nolan et al. 2005).

A full neurological examination may be helpful. However, for the purposes of rapid assessment of responsiveness in the acutely ill patients, the AVPU scale is commonly used.

A – alert;
V – responds to voice;
P – responds to pain;
U – unresponsive.

Blood glucose should always be monitored to exclude hypoglycaemia as a cause for change in the level of consciousness. Give 50 mL or 10% glucose solution if the level is below 3 mmol. Give further doses as needed to correct the blood glucose.

E – Exposure

Exposure refers to the necessity for a full visual physical inspection and examination of the patient. For example, there may not be an obvious sign of bleeding or of injury; therefore, it is important to examine the patient from head to toe, front and back. Maintain the patient's dignity at all times.

REVIEW OF LEARNING

❑ Most cardiac arrests are avoidable if recognised and treated early.
❑ Most cardiac arrests are associated with ACS or related symptoms.
❑ Recognising the acutely ill patient requires skill and knowledge of how to perform a systematic clinical assessment and identify priorities.
❑ Assessment of a patient whose condition is deteriorating must include Airway, Breathing, Circulation, Disability and Exposure.
❑ Track and trigger systems can provide evidence of a deterioration in a patient's condition.
❑ Healthcare professionals should be aware of local procedures for summoning expert assistance based on track and trigger scores.

Case study

Helen Browning is a 72-year-old woman admitted to the ward for a chest infection. She has been on the ward for 12 hours and routine observations and blood tests have been done. She is now complaining of feeling unwell and short of breath. Her observations indicate that her respiratory rate is 30–34 breaths/min, pulse rate 95 beats/min and blood pressure 95/40 mm Hg.

   Without reading the text, write down **what further assessment is required**?

A – Speak to her. If she responds appropriately, it is evident that her airway is open. If she does not respond, assess the airway further looking, listening and feeling for air movement, noisy breathing or any other signs of airway obstruction.

B – Count her respiratory rate and compare this to the track and trigger system available on the ward. Call for help if needed. Look for other signs of breathing problems or difficulties. Start oxygen with a non-rebreathing mask at 10–15 L/min. Assess her oxygenation with a pulse oximeter

C – Measure and record her heart rate and blood pressure and compare this to the track and trigger system available on the ward. Call for help, if needed. Be sure Helen has IV access and prepare to give IV fluid. Assess for other signs of cardiovascular problems (e.g. cool hands and feet, increased capillary refill time, cyanosis). Start ECG monitoring.

D – Do a quick neurological assessment using AVPU. Check blood glucose and give 50 mL of 10% glucose solution if the level is below 3 mmol.

E – Look for any other worrying signs.

CONCLUSION

Recognising and responding to the early signs and symptoms in the patient who is critically ill and at risk of a cardiac arrest demands skilled systematic assessment of vital functions in order to intervene appropriately. Nurses at the bedside are most likely to identify this group of vulnerable patients and therefore their assessment and actions will be of vital significance in preventing many avoidable deaths.

REFERENCES

Albarran, J.W. & Tagney, J. (eds) (2007) *Chest Pain: Advanced Assessment and Management Skills.* Blackwell Publishing, Oxford.

Arntz, H.R., Bossaert, L. & Filippatos, G.S. (2005) European Resuscitation Council guidelines for resuscitation 2005. Section 4: adult advanced life support. *Resuscitation* **67** (suppl I), 39–86.

Dellinger, R.P., Levy, M.M., Carlet, J.M. *et al.* (2008) Surviving sepsis campaign: international guidelines for management of severe sepsis and septic shock: 2008. *Critical Care Medicine* **36** (1), 296–327.

Guyton, A.C. & Hall, J.E. (2005) *Textbook of Medical Physiology,* 11th edn. Saunders, Philadelphia.

Harrison, G.A., Jacques, T.C., Kilborn, G. & McLaws, M.L. (2005) The prevalence of recordings of the signs of critical conditions and emergency responses in hospital wards – the SOCCER study. *Resuscitation* **65**, 149–57.

Jowett, N.I. & Thompson, D.R. (2003) *Comprehensive Coronary Care,* 3rd edn. Baillière Tindall, Edinburgh.

Kause, J., Smith, G., Prytherch, D. *et al.* (2004) A comparison of antecedents to cardiac arrests, deaths and emergency intensive care admissions in Australia and New Zealand, and the United Kingdom – the ACADEMIA study. *Resuscitation* **62**, 275–82.

McGaughey, J., Alderdice, F., Fowler, R., Kapila, A., Mayhew, A. & Moutray, M. (2007) Outreach and early warning systems (EWS) for the prevention of intensive care admission and death of critically ill adult patients on general hospital wards. *Cochrane Database of Systematic Reviews* 3, CD 00 55 29.

National Confidential Enquiry into Patient Outcome and Death (2005) *An Acute Problem?* National Confidential Enquiry into Patient Outcome and Death, London.

National Institute for Clinical Excellence (2007) *Recognition of and Response to Acute Illness in Adults in Hospital.* Available online at: www.nice.org.uk.

Nolan, J.P., Deakin, C.D., Soar, J., Bottiger, B.W. & Smith, G. (2005) European Resuscitation Council guidelines for resuscitation 2005. Section 4: adult advanced life support. *Resuscitation* **67** (suppl I), 39–86.

Peberdy, M.A., Kaye, W., Ornato, J.P. *et al.* (2003) Cardiopulmonary resuscitation of adults in the hospital: a report of 14720 cardiac arrests from the National Registry of Cardiopulmonary Resuscitation. *Resuscitation* **58**, 297–308.

Resuscitation Council UK (2006) *Advanced Life Support Course Provider Manual,* 5th edn. Resuscitation Council UK, London.

Smith, G.B. (2003) *ALERT. A Multiprofessional Course in Care of the Acutely Ill,* 2nd edn. University of Portsmouth, Portsmouth.

Smith, G.B., Osgood, V.M. & Crane, S., for the ALERT Course Development Group (2002) ALERTTM – a multiprofessional training course in the care of the acutely ill adult patient. *Resuscitation* **52**, 281–6.

Smith, G.B., Prytherch, D.R., Schmidt, P.E. & Featherstone, P.I. (2008) Review and performance evaluation of aggregate weighted 'track and trigger' systems. *Resuscitation* **77**, 170–79.

4 Resuscitation Equipment

Una McKay

INTRODUCTION

The best possible chance of patient survival following a cardiac arrest in a clinical environment can be given only if the arrest is promptly recognised and responded to by staff who have received appropriate training. To facilitate the rapid resuscitation of any patient, provision should be made in all clinical areas to have immediate access to appropriate equipment and drugs (Resuscitation Council UK 2004). The choice of resuscitation equipment should be defined by the hospital Resuscitation Committee and may be influenced to some degree by specialised local requirements. Most general hospitals will organise their resuscitation equipment onto a trolley that is known as the 'cardiac arrest' or 'crash' trolley. Other hospitals or departments may assemble their equipment in the form of a 'grab bag' or a wall-mounted board or box. Whichever system is used, it is important that the resuscitation equipment and defibrillators are standardised throughout an organisation, so that any attending cardiac arrest or emergency team member will be presented with the same system regardless of the ward or department they are responding to. Where possible, resuscitation equipment should be single use and latex free (Resuscitation Council UK 2004).

AIMS

This chapter considers equipment that is commonly used in a respiratory or cardiac arrest situation and outlines considerations regarding the maintenance of equipment.

LEARNING OUTCOMES

By the end of the chapter, the reader will be able to:

❑ list *essential resuscitation equipment* for dealing with a patient's airway, breathing and circulation;
❑ appreciate the way in which *cardiac arrest equipment may be organised*;
❑ appreciate *other miscellaneous equipment* that may be required during a resuscitation attempt;
❑ outline their *individual responsibilities* with regard to resuscitation equipment.

RESUSCITATION EQUIPMENT

The Resuscitation Council UK (2004) provides a list of recommended minimum equipment for in-hospital adult resuscitation as follows.

Airway and breathing equipment (see Figures 4.1 and 4.2)

- Pocket masks with oxygen port;
- Self-inflating bag-valve with oxygen reservoir and tubing – ideally, single use or if not, then equipment with a suitable filter;
- Clear facemasks, sizes 3, 4 and 5;
- Oropharyngeal airways, sizes 2, 3 and 4;
- Nasopharyngeal airways, sizes 6 and 7;
- Yankaeur suckers;

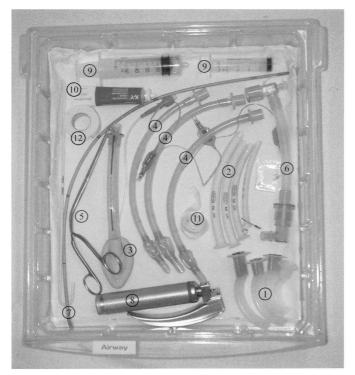

Index of equipment

1. Guedel airways
2. Nasopharyngeal airways
3. LMA
4. Endotracheal tubes (oral and cuffed)
5. McGill forceps
6. Catheter mount with swivel connector
7. Gum elastic bougie
8. Laryngoscope with curved blade (spare laryngoscope with blades should also be available)
9. Syringes (10 ml and 50 ml)
10. Lubricant
11. 1″ (2.5 cm) ribbon gauze or tape
12. Micropore

Figure 4.1 Airway drawer of a cardiac arrest trolley (adult).

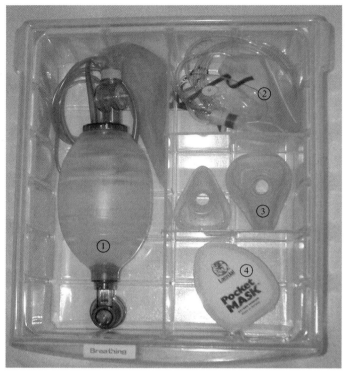

Index of equipment

1. Self-inflating resuscitation bag with oxygen reservoir and oxygen tubing
2. Clear oxygen facemask with reservoir bag
3. Clear facemask to be attached to (1)
4. Pocket mask used to deliver assisted breaths in the unconscious patient

Figure 4.2 Breathing drawer of a cardiac arrest trolley (adult).

- Portable suction unit or manual suction device;
- Endotracheal suction catheters, sizes 12 and 14;
- Laryngeal mask airway (sizes 4 and 5) or combitube (small);
- Magill forceps;
- Endotracheal tubes – oral and cuffed, sizes 6, 7 and 8;
- Catheter mount;
- Gum elastic bougie;
- Lubricating jelly;
- Laryngoscopes (ideally two, with standard and long blades);
- Spare laryngoscope bulbs and batteries;
- 1″ (2.5 cm) ribbon gauze/tape for securing tracheal tubes;
- Scissors;
- Syringes – 20 and 50 mL;
- Clear oxygen mask with reservoir (non-rebreathing) bag;
- Oxygen cylinder/supply;
- Cylinder key.

Circulation equipment

- Defibrillator (shock advisory module and/or pacing facility to be determined by local policy);
- ECG electrodes;
- Defibrillation gel pads or self-adhesive defibrillator pads (preferred);
- Selection of needles and syringes;
- Intravenous (IV) cannulaes 18 gauge and 14 gauge;
- Cannulae fixing dressings and tape;
- Seldinger wire central line kit;
- IV infusion sets;
- Arterial blood gas syringe;
- Torniquet;
- 0.9% sodium chloride – 1000 mL × 2.

Drugs

Immediately available pre-filled syringes:

- adrenaline/epinephrine 1 mg (1:10 000) × 4;
- atropine 3 mg × 1;
- amiodarone 300 mg × 1.

Other readily available drugs:

- adenosine 6 mg × 10;
- adrenaline (epinephrine) 1:1000 × 2;
- adrenalin (epinephrine) 1 mg (1:10 000) × 4;
- amiodarone 300 mg × 1;
- calcium chloride 10 mL of 100 mg/mL × 1;
- chlorphenamine 10 mg × 2;
- glucose 10% 500 mL × 1;
- hydrocortisone 100 mg × 2;
- lidocaine 100 mg × 1;
- magnesium sulphate 50% solution 2 g (4 mL) × 1;
- midazolam 10 mg × 1;
- naloxone 400 µg × 2;
- normal saline 10 mL ampoules;
- potassium chloride for injection;
- sodium bicarbonate 8.4% – 50 mL × 1.

Other medications

- Salbutamol (5 mg × 2) and ipratropium bromide (500 µg × 2) nebules;
- Nebuliser device and mask;
- GTN spray;
- Aspirin 300 mg.

Additional items that should be readily available

- Sharps box and clinical waste bag;
- Large scissors;

- Alcohol wipes;
- Blood sample bottles;
- Razors;
- Audit form;
- Clock;
- Gloves/goggles/aprons, sliding sheet or similar manual handling device.

Access will also be required for equipment that is not necessarily needed immediately during the resuscitation but will certainly be required post-arrest, such as a blood pressure measuring device, a pulse oximeter and a 12-lead electrocardiograph (ECG) machine.

Equipment for the primary care environment

Due to the specific nature of the primary care environment, a separate document outlines the minimal equipment that should be available in such a setting (Resuscitation Council UK 2001). This is basically a scaled-down version of the standard equipment noted above and takes into consideration the possibility of very few personnel being available to deal with the cardiac arrest. In many situations, there may simply be one person to deal with the arrest.

Equipment for the management of paediatric cardiopulmonary arrest

Much of the equipment required to manage paediatric cardiac arrest reflects that use in adult resuscitation. The major difference is in the size range of equipment that needs to be available as paediatric patients range from zero to 16 years of age, hence a much wider selection of everything, from airway adjuncts to vascular devices is required. A suggested list of equipment is provided by the Resuscitation Council UK (2003). One notable piece of equipment that is suggested is a type of profile chart such as the Broselow tape[TM] or Oakley chart. These charts aid the estimation of children's weight in the emergency situation.

THE CARDIAC ARREST TROLLEY

Cardiac arrest trolleys (or other system) should ideally be located in every clinical ward and department. A list of the contents of the trolley should be available and some kind of system established to ensure that the trolley content has been checked on a daily or weekly basis (and immediately after use). It should be noted that it is the responsibility of every healthcare professional to be familiar with the layout and contents of their organisation's trolley or system. One of the best ways to ensure familiarity is to regularly get involved in checking the trolley. Staff who carry out equipment checks should be accountable for the integrity and functioning of the equipment, and checklists should be signed as proof of compliance (Dyson & Smith 2002). Locum or agency staff should always be orientated to the location of the emergency equipment.

Cardiac arrest trolleys are often laid out according to the ABC of resuscitation. For example, a trolley containing three or four drawers can be used with the individual drawers being labelled 'Airway', 'Breathing' and 'Circulation' and possibly a fourth drawer for miscellaneous items. Most resuscitation trolleys will accommodate an oxygen cylinder and suction unit on the side with a defibrillator often being stored on top. It must be remembered that mechanical equipment such as suction and the defibrillator will generally be plugged into the mains electricity socket to be kept on charge and as such it will need to be unplugged before quickly moving the trolley.

Equipment for managing the airway

Often the airway and breathing are considered to be the same thing and equipment such as a pocket mask may be found in the airway drawer as opposed to the breathing drawer. Figure 4.1 is an example of how an 'airway drawer' may be set out. With this particular type of trolley system, each drawer can actually be removed from the trolley, so the airway drawer, for example, may be passed up to the head of the patient to allow the healthcare professional managing the airway easier access to the equipment they are likely to require. The drawers also have a plastic lid-type cover to them (not shown), which works well in preventing the accumulation of dust on the equipment.

Oropharyngeal airways

- This is often referred to as a *Guedel airway*™ (see Figure 4.1, item 1).
- It is a plastic, curved tube, with a reinforced section and flange at the oral end. The reinforced section is a bite block and is designed to sit between the teeth. The remainder of the tube fits between the tongue and posterior pharyngeal wall.
- The oral airway can be used only in patients who are unconscious or sedated with no gag reflex. It will cause gagging or straining in a patient whose reflex responses are intact. Such a patient may be a suitable candidate for a nasopharyngeal airway.
- The oropharyngeal airway comes in a range of sizes to fit newborns up to large adults.
- For guidelines on sizing and insertion, see Chapter 9.

Nasopharyngeal airways

- Designed to help maintain a patent airway. They are indicated in the patient who is not deeply unconscious and therefore unable to tolerate an oropharyngeal airway, yet needs a simple adjunct to help maintain airway patency.
- Nasopharyngeal airways are soft, flexible plastic tubes with an angular end and a trumpet-shaped end.
- They may be particularly useful in patients with maxillofacial injuries or in situations where it is impossible to open the patient's mouth (clenched or wired jaws, trismus).
- This device is best avoided in a patient with a base-of-skull fracture for fear of intracranial insertion.
- For guidelines on sizing and insertion, see Chapter 9.

Laryngeal mask airway

The laryngeal mask airway (LMA) is an adjunctive airway composed of a wide-bore tube with an elliptical inflatable cuff that, when inflated, provides a seal around the laryngeal opening (see Figure 4.1, item 3). The LMA is an extremely reliable device that can be used during a resuscitation attempt by nurses and other paramedical staff who may not be skilled in endotracheal intubation (Anonymous 1994). It is important, as with any piece of equipment, that the operator has undergone the necessary training and assessment procedures as outlined by their place of work. For guidelines on sizing and insertion, see Chapter 9.

Endotracheal tube

- Designed to offer full protection in securing the patient's airway. Considered to be the 'gold standard' in maintaining an airway.
- The cuffed tube is inserted directly into the trachea under clear and direct vision using a laryngoscope.
- Prior to inflation of the cuff, the operator checks for correct tube placement by auscultation of the lungs with a stethoscope.
- The endotracheal tube (ETT) may be attached directly to a ventilation device such as a bag-valve system with or without oxygen attached.
- A fine-bore suction catheter may be inserted through the ETT to remove secretions, etc. from the lower airways.
- The ETT is an alternative route for drug delivery in the event of IV access not being achieved.

Magill forceps

- Forceps with long angled levers designed to assist in removing objects or foreign bodies from the patient's airway, for example a dislodged denture plate.
- They may also be used in assisting intubation.

Catheter mount with swivel connector

- Designed to fit between the end connection port of an ETT, LMA or combitube (see Chapter 9) and the bag-valve ventilation system.
- The catheter mount gives an extra bit of leeway between the bag and any tube, generally resulting in less possibility of dislodging a tube.
- An added bonus is that a port on top of the catheter mount will allow the passage of a soft suction catheter down through the tube to remove any secretions. This can be performed without having to disconnect the bag from the tube on each occasion, hence reducing the risk of dislodging the tube.

Introducers

- Two types of introducers are shown in Figure 4.1, item 7. There is a rigid introducer (or stylet) and a gum elastic flexible introducer, known as a bougie.
- During intubation, the rigid introducer may be used inside an ETT to alter the natural curvature of the tube depending on the patient's airway anatomy.
- The bougie can also aid in difficult intubation but this tends to be inserted into the airway first and the ETT would then be slipped over the bougie and into the correct place using the bougie as a guide.

Laryngoscope

- The laryngoscope (see Figure 4.1, item 8) is a device generally used for intubation and to give direct clear vision of a patient's oropharynx. It may have other uses, such as providing a light source during the removal of foreign material.
- During daily or weekly checking of the trolley, the blade of the laryngoscope should be pulled up to a 90° angle and locked in place to assess the brightness of the light source and battery function.
- Different sized blades are recommended although for most adult patients, a size 3 Macintosh blade will suffice.
- It is a good idea to have a second laryngoscope on the trolley in the event of failure of the first.
- Spare batteries and bulbs (if it is not of a fibreoptic type) should always be available on the trolley, as well as different types of blade, i.e. standard and long.

Miscellaneous

There are other things which will be necessary in airway management, such as:

- lubricating jelly – to assist in nasopharyngeal, LMA or ETT insertion;
- tape or ribbon gauze – to tie in or secure an airway device such as an LMA or ETT;
- syringe – airway devices such as the ETT and LMA will require inflation with air. An LMA, depending on size, may require up to 40 mL of air to be inserted.

More information on the use of airway equipment may be found in Chapter 9.

Equipment for managing breathing

Figure 4.2 is an example of how the 'breathing drawer' of a cardiac arrest trolley may be laid out. In some departments, the bag-valve-mask system may be found readily attached to the oxygen and in a more accessible location, where it can be seen hooked on the drip stand. However, if it is located in the drawer as indicated below, it is less likely to accumulate dust.

Bag-valve system

This system is often still referred to as the Ambu-Bag™ as Ambu was one of the first manufacturers to make the device readily available. It consists of a self-inflating bag and a one-way non-rebreathing valve. When the bag is squeezed, the air is delivered to the patient's lungs via the one-way valve. On releasing the squeeze, the bag self-inflates with room air that enters via an inlet at the opposite end of the bag. When oxygen becomes available, a reservoir bag should be attached to this inlet and the oxygen flow set at 10–15 L/min. The patient's exhaled air is released back into the atmosphere by the one-way valve and does not contaminate the contents of the bag. The bag-valve device may be used with a facemask, an LMA, an endotracheal tube or a combitube (Resuscitation Council UK 2006).

Pocket mask

- The pocket mask is a facemask that allows mouth-to-mask ventilation of the patient (see Figure 4.2, item 4).
- It is available with or without an inlet that allows additional oxygen to be attached. Preferably one with an oxygen inlet should be used in the hospital setting.
- The pocket mask is available in one size for adults and will allow a good seal in most casualties.
- For guidelines on sizing and insertion, see Chapter 9.

Non-rebreather oxygen masks

- For the patient who is spontaneously breathing, an oxygen mask should be available (see Figure 4.2, item 2).
- The non-rebreather oxygen mask has a reservoir bag attached, allowing an oxygen concentration of about 85% when delivered at a flow rate of 10–15 L/min.

More information on the use of ventilation equipment may be found in Chapter 9.

Equipment for managing the circulation

IV connectors and three-way taps

- A selection of connectors is necessary for any IV infusions that may be commenced.
- Three-way taps are often connected between a giving set and the patient's IV access so that a syringe can be attached, allowing boluses of saline to be drawn from the bag and pushed into the IV line following administration of any drug bolus.

Giving sets and air inlets

- A giving set may be required for the administration of IV fluid.
- Depending on the IV fluid container type, an air inlet (wide-bore needles with special filter) may need to be inserted into the container to increase the rate of fluid administration.

Selection of hypodermic needles

- Several needles may be required for the drawing up of cardiac arrest drugs that are sometimes not available in pre-filled syringes. They may also be required for drawing up saline boluses if the method suggested above is not used.
- Blood gas syringes may be located in this drawer also.

Razors, 12-lead ECG electrodes and normal ECG monitoring electrodes

- It is always useful to have several razors available in case the patient's chest is very hairy, resulting in ECG electrodes that fail to adhere properly to the chest wall.

- The ECG electrodes should be replaced on the trolley regularly as once removed from their packet, the gel within the electrode may dry out and result in an electrode not sticking to the chest wall in an emergency.

IV cannulae
Early access to the circulation is important in cardiac arrest so that drugs can be administered quickly. A selection of large-bore cannulae should be available.

IV cannulae dressing
In an emergency, normal surgical tape can be used to secure a cannula in place but having a proper IV cannulae dressing will offer extra security against any IV access accidentally being dislodged.

Water/normal saline for injection
Saline boluses may be given directly from a bag of saline connected to the IV line by a giving set. However, if this option is not employed then normal 20-mL ampoules are required. Water for injection may be necessary for drawing up some types of drugs.

Scissors
A pair of heavy-duty scissors may be required to cut through some types of clothing and gain access to the chest so that defibrillation can be performed quickly.

Tourniquet
Gaining IV access is often difficult in a cardiac arrest situation. In an emergency, one member of the team may use his or her hands to form a tourniquet around the patient's limb whilst another team member may insert the cannula. However, this does not offer an even tourniquet pressure and therefore use of a proper tourniquet is more desirable.

Gauze and surgical tape
- Gauze pads may be required to cover any bleeding sites, for example following blood gas analysis or removal of a cannula.
- Surgical tape may be used to secure gauze in place or to secure an airway device, for example an ETT.

Further information on IV access and drug delivery can be found in Chapter 12 and more information on ECG monitoring and defibrillation may be found in Chapters 10 and 11.

Drugs and fluids
Drugs and fluids may be considered part of the equipment needed for circulation and many hospitals will have specific 'cardiac arrest drug boxes'. These are often separated down further into 'first-line' and 'second-line' drugs. The list recommended by the Resuscitation Council UK (2004) is very comprehensive, particularly the section on 'other readily available drugs'. This could be interpreted as 'second-line' drugs and whilst desirable, it is not absolutely necessary to keep all

of these on the trolley, particularly if space is limited. In this case, the second-line drugs should be kept together in an appropriate location that is easily and rapidly accessible.

IV fluids
- There has been lengthy debate regarding the best type of fluid to be given in emergency situations. Most cardiac arrest trolleys should stock both a crystalloid (such as 0.9% normal saline) and a colloid (such as gelofusin).
- A bag of 5% dextrose is often kept on the trolley as, if pre-filled syringes are not available, this is the medium generally used if diluting the drug amiodarone.

Pre-filled drug syringes
There are two different pre-filled drug systems in general use in the UK – the Min-I-Jet™ system and the Aurum™ system. See Chapter 12 for advice on the assembly and use of these systems.

Miscellaneous equipment
A miscellaneous drawer is useful for storing essential equipment that may be too bulky or cumbersome or just take up a lot of space in one of the other drawers, for example spare oxygen masks, laryngoscope bulbs and spares.

Suction catheters
- Any suction device is likely to have a rigid suction catheter already attached to it but several spare catheters should be on the trolley.
- A selection of fine-bore flexible catheters should also be available.
- These catheters may be more appropriately placed in the airway drawer, depending on available space.

Spare canister for the suction apparatus
As it is possible that arrests may occur sequentially with no time for restocking of the trolley, it is most useful to have at least one spare of everything.

Gloves/goggles/aprons
The use of personal protective equipment during a cardiac arrest situation is strongly recommended, particularly the use of gloves as contact with body fluids is very likely.

Defibrillation gel pads
Often the defibrillation gel pads are stored on top of the defibrillator, so that they are immediately obvious to the operator. However, the defibrillator, when attached to the mains in charging mode, will generate a very small amount of warmth and this may dry out the gel pads. Storing them elsewhere is therefore recommended (see Chapter 11).

INDIVIDUAL RESPONSIBILITIES
Every healthcare practitioner has a responsibility to be familiar with cardiac arrest equipment. Practical training in the use of resuscitation equipment is likely to be

available through the hospital Resuscitation Officer. Whilst familiarity is required by all healthcare professionals, training in the actual use of a piece of equipment may not be appropriate; for example, using a laryngoscope and ETT to intubate a patient is a very specialist skill.

Following a resuscitation attempt, it is important that the cardiac arrest trolley or system is replenished almost immediately in case a further cardiac arrest occurs in a short time frame. Whilst single use equipment is recommended during resuscitation, equipment such as LMAs or laryngoscopes may be auto-clavable and hence policies and procedures for cleaning and replenishment of equipment should be adhered to.

It is always worth considering what would happen in the event of equipment failure and where alternative equipment may be found. Faulty equipment, or any problems experienced by staff which place patients at risk should be documented and reported using a critical incident reporting system so that the matter is fully investigated and action is taken to prevent the same problem from occurring again (Dyson & Smith 2002).

REVIEW OF LEARNING
- ❏ Resuscitation equipment should be available to all departments and wards.
- ❏ This should include airway, breathing and circulation equipment and drugs.
- ❏ The equipment should be organised systematically for easy access and use.
- ❏ All resuscitation equipment should be checked daily and following arrests.
- ❏ Every healthcare practitioner should be familiar with the cardiac arrest equipment.

Case study

Review and consider the answers to the following questions.

- Are you familiar with and able to identify the contents of your cardiac arrest trolley or system?
- Do you know where to seek further training in your organisation?
- Do you know how to replenish the trolley after it has been used?
- Do you know which equipment is disposable and which needs to be cleaned and disinfected, either locally or centrally?
- Do you know what to do in the event of equipment failure?

There are no answers provided, as you need to know the system that is particular to your individual organisation. If you are uncertain on any aspect then you have a professional responsibility to seek clarity.

CONCLUSION
It is imperative that every healthcare practitioner is familiar with any equipment that they may have to use in an emergency. A cardiac arrest is almost always a stressful situation and lack of knowledge or familiarity with equipment and procedures will only increase the pressures of the event and is likely to delay

appropriate interventions for the patient. Ultimately, this decreases the chance of a successful resuscitation.

REFERENCES

Anonymous (1994) The use of the laryngeal mask airway by nurses during cardiopulmonary resuscitation – results of a multicentre trial. *Anaesthesia* **49** (1), 3–7.

Dyson, E. & Smith, G.B. (2002) Common faults in resuscitation equipment – guidelines for checking equipment and drugs used in adult cardiopulmonary resuscitation. *Resuscitation* **55**, 137–49.

Resuscitation Council UK (2001) *Cardiopulmonary Resuscitation. Guidance for Clinical Practice and Training in Primary Care.* Resuscitation Council UK, London.

Resuscitation Council UK (2003) *Suggested Equipment for the Management of Paediatric Cardiopulmonary Arrest (0–16 Years) (Excluding Resuscitation at Birth) Resuscitation.* Resuscitation Council UK, London.

Resuscitation Council UK (2004) *Recommended Minimum Equipment for In-Hospital Adult Resuscitation.* Resuscitation Council UK, London.

Resuscitation Council UK (2006) *Advanced Life Support Course Provider Manual*, 5th edn. Resuscitation Council UK, London.

Chain of Survival

5

Ben King

INTRODUCTION

Effective resuscitation is dependent on a number of different interventions happening within as short a time as possible. From the first moment when a bystander recognises and confirms a cardiac arrest right the way through until sophisticated management strategies are being considered in a specialist unit, the team's speed of response is of the utmost importance.

The members of the team are similar to a chain in that they are totally dependent on each other and if one link is not functioning, the chain breaks and teamwork fails. The 'Chain of Survival' therefore represents the combination of the individual components involved in the management of an emergency.

This idea of linking the basic resuscitation of first responders to the advanced life support may be seen as common sense. However, a great deal of time and money has been spent seeking to improve all aspects of the system and how those involved work together (Cummins *et al.* 1991).

AIMS

This chapter describes the development of the 'Chain of Survival' concept, its implementation and its relevance to current resuscitation practice.

LEARNING OUTCOMES

At the end of the chapter, the reader will be able to:

❏ describe the *links* in the Chain of Survival;
❏ understand the *rationale* for developing the Chain of Survival;
❏ describe how the Chain of Survival *operates in both community and hospital settings*.

The four links in the Chain of Survival are shown in Figure 5.1.

DEVELOPMENT OF THE CHAIN OF SURVIVAL

The concept of the Chain of Survival has not changed significantly since it was first described even though individual components such as basic life support (BLS) and defibrillation have been refined and redirected.

The need to link the efforts of those responding to an emergency was described as far back as the 1960s. Its genesis was based on the pre-hospital setting to deal

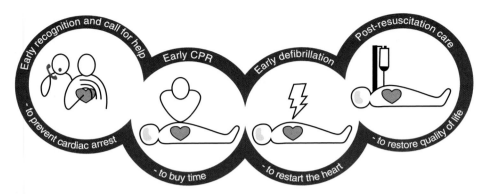

Figure 5.1   Chain of Survival.

with the problem of sudden cardiac death (SCD) in the community. Peter Safar recognised the need to link basic cardiopulmonary resuscitation (CPR), whose aim was to 'buy time', to advanced life support (ALS), whose aim was to re-store spontaneous circulation (Newman 1998). This message was developed by Mary Newman of the Citizen Foundation, who introduced the chain of survival metaphor in 1987 (Newman 1989). By the mid-1980s, the importance of early de-fibrillation had been established and as such became a component of the chain in its own right.

The Chain of Survival has the following links:

- early recognition and call for help – to prevent cardiac arrest;
- early CPR – to buy time;
- early defibrillation – to re-start the heart;
- post-resuscitation care – to restore the quality of life.

IMPLEMENTATION OF THE CHAIN OF SURVIVAL

Early recognition and call for help

The call to summon expert help and emergency equipment will either be a 999/112 call in the UK community setting or a resuscitation team call in hospital. This will ensure that advanced airway/breathing equipment, a defibrillator and emergency drugs are dispatched at the earliest opportunity.

Telephoning for assistance relies on the first rescuer assessing the casualty, ac-curately recognising the situation and responding by summoning help.

Early access will not be achieved if the rescuer:

- chooses not to approach the casualty – real or perceived risks;
- fails to recognise the serious nature of the situation;
- does not know how to access help – inadequate training.

This link aims to promote prevention of in-hospital cardiac arrests using the strategies outlined in Chapter 3 and out-of-hospital cardiac arrests by encour-aging the public to seek expert help more quickly via the emergency services.

Particular emphasis for the public is risks of cardiovascular disease and chest pain.

Early CPR

Chest compressions achieve only 25–30% of normal cardiac output (Resuscitation Council UK 2005). Thus, CPR delivers considerably less oxygen to vital organs than they normally receive; so it cannot prevent organ damage over an extended period of time. This reinforces the need for early access to expert help in both the hospital and community settings.

The options open to the rescuer with regard to *how* to commence CPR will vary depending on the availability of equipment and expert assistance.

The purpose of CPR is to effectively perfuse the body's vital organs such as the heart and brain during the period of absent circulation. It will rarely restore spontaneous circulation on its own, which is why the next link in the chain is defibrillation.

Early defibrillation

CPR is a means of 'buying time' for all casualties prior to the arrival of the defibrillator. However, if the defibrillator is immediately available, for example in a coronary care unit or ambulance, it should be used without delay. Approximately, 30% of in-hospital cardiac arrests (Gwinnutt *et al.* 2000) and 80% of those out of hospital (Eisenberg & Mengert 2001) have shockable rhythms as their first recorded rhythms (see Chapter 11 for further details).

Post-resuscitation care

Many more lives have been saved by the application of the first three links of the Chain of Survival but effective and timely ALS will influence not only survival but also the quality of life. The interventions undertaken by a hospital cardiac arrest team or paramedics in the out-of-hospital setting will include intubation to protect the airway, securing intravenous access and administering cardiac arrest drugs. Whilst this is happening, it is also essential to assess the casualty's clinical history for potentially reversible causes and ensure that CPR remains effective.

Continued resuscitation or post-resuscitation care aims to stabilise the patient during the vulnerable time after spontaneous circulation has been restored.

DEBATE SURROUNDING THE CHAIN OF SURVIVAL

'Phone First' or 'CPR First'

The question of whether the *lone rescuer* should initiate CPR or should first phone for help proved difficult to answer. If defibrillation is of such importance then access to help should come first. The counterargument ran that CPR provided oxygenation to the brain and may actually restore spontaneous circulation in some patients.

It has been established that for those patients suspected of sustaining a cardiac arrest that is cardiac in origin, the call for the emergency services should precede CPR. This is due to the fact that CPR will slow down but not prevent the deterioration of ventricular fibrillation (VF) to fine VF and then asystole so early

Table 5.1 Cardiac arrests when one minute of CPR should be completed first.

Cause of cardiac arrest	Primary system involved
Submersion/near drowning	Airway/breathing
Arrest associated with trauma	Airway
Drug overdose	Respiratory depression
Children (who are not at risk of arrhythmias)	Airway/breathing

defibrillation is essential. In a cardiac arrest caused by hypoxia (a) the rhythm is less likely to be shockable (so a defibrillator is less useful) and (b) CPR may reverse the hypoxia, thus treating the cause and restoring perfusion.

Rescuers encountering a casualty who they suspect has collapsed due to a hypoxic cause should carry out one minute of CPR prior to phoning for help. Obviously, if two or more rescuers are present, one can get expert help while the other commences resuscitation.

Cause of cardiac arrest

Due to the prevalence of coronary artery disease, the rescuer encountering an adult with absent sign of life should assume the cause is cardiac in origin, usually an acute coronary syndrome causing a tachyarrhythmia. In the absence of other clues, this is a statistically safe assumption to make (Phone First). Evidence that might suggest a non-cardiac cause would include signs of severe trauma, the possibility of near drowning or evidence of a potential drug over dose (CPR First).

The situation for children is different due to the extremely small risk of a cardiac arrest having a primary cardiac cause. It is estimated that paediatric arrests will present in shockable rhythms in approximately 10% of cases (Young & Siedel 1999) compared to 80% for adults (Eisenberg & Mengert 2001).

The rescuer encountering a collapsed child/infant should assume the cause is hypoxia, i.e. non-cardiac in origin (CPR First). There may be rare occasions where the child is suspected of having a primary cardiac cause for his or her collapse. These include, the child has known cardiac disease, a very sudden, very unexpected collapse, particularly during exercise or the possibility of electrocution (Phone First).

The situations in Table 5.1 are examples of when the lone rescuer should initially complete a full minute of CPR before leaving the casualty to phone for help.

HOW THE CHAIN OF SURVIVAL FUNCTIONS IN PRACTICE

This can be divided into pre-hospital and in-hospital settings.

The pre-hospital setting

There is continuing evidence supporting the importance of the chain working as a single unit rather than as separate entities. Researchers have clearly demonstrated that survival is severely diminished if a single link fails (Cummins *et al.* 1991).

Table 5.2 Effects of minimal delay.

Collapse to CPR	Collapse to defibrillation	
	<10 min	>10 min
<5 min	37% survival	7% survival
>5 min	20% survival	0% survival

How the chain may break

- Access – this may be delayed if the casualty is in an unsafe environment, is not found or if bystanders are either unwilling or lacking confidence to get involved.
- CPR – a layperson finding a casualty may phone for help very rapidly but then fail to provide effective CPR. Survival to discharge from out-of-hospital cardiac arrest doubles if CPR is started within 4 minutes (Larsen *et al.* 1993). Effective CPR is associated with a greater incidence of the first recorded rhythm being VF (Dowie *et al.* 2003).
- Defibrillation – even if a rapid phone call for help and bystander CPR do occur immediately, defibrillation may be delayed by a number of factors such as traffic and distance.

The success of the chain in the pre-hospital setting is demonstrated in examples where limited equipment is available, such as on aeroplanes (Page *et al.* 2000), railway stations (Davies 2002), in general practitioner surgeries (Colquhoun 2002) and in Las Vegas casinos (Valenzuela *et al.* 2000). In all these settings, the time from collapse to being found was short (early access); CPR was started promptly (early CPR) and they are all settings where shock advisory defibrillators were provided (early defibrillation).

Compared to the first three links, the introduction of drugs has had only limited impact (Mitchell *et al.* 2000).

Table 5.2 illustrates that where either early CPR or early defibrillation occurs, the survival is considerably less than if both occur with minimal delay (Cummins *et al.* 1985).

The ideal provision for out-of-hospital cardiac arrests includes:

- large percentage of the population know how to summon emergency help;
- high proportion of the public trained to recognise and respond to cardiac arrest;
- public access defibrillators and first responder schemes in place;
- facility for rapid transfer of patient to critical care setting.

The in-hospital setting

When an inpatient has a cardiac arrest, his or her chances of surviving to discharge from hospital are approximately one in seven (Gwinnutt *et al.* 2000).

In the hospital environment, early access and early CPR should be achieved by appropriate staff training. In addition to this, many nurses and doctors will be available to defibrillate the casualty and provide ALS. At first glance, the Chain of

Survival looks very strong so it is of concern that the overall in-hospital survival is only 17%.

Underlying factors for this survival rate include the following.

- The degree of illness (co-morbidity) present in the in-hospital population. Compared to the general population, this group is more likely to be suffering from chronic disease. It has been shown that the greater the degree of chronic disease, the lower the chances of survival from cardiac arrest (Ambury *et al.* 2000).
- The first presenting cardiac rhythm, which is likely to be non-shockable. These cardiac arrest rhythms have lower survival rates than VF/VT arrests and are the presenting rhythm in two thirds of in-hospital cardiac arrests (Gwinnutt *et al.* 2000).
- The patient is very likely to deteriorate either gradually or dramatically over a period of time. At the end of this period of inadequate ventilation or circulatory failure, the patient will be suffering some degree of hypoxia and multiorgan failure. Cardiac arrest in this instance will be more difficult to reverse.

The concept of the Chain of Survival has demonstrated that each link on its own has limited benefit unless all the links in the chain are present. When dealing with the sick or deteriorating in-hospital patient, it could be considered that there is a 'chain of responsibility'. When a critical incident occurs, it is rarely found to be the fault of one individual but is more commonly proved to be a failure in the system (DH 1998). Evidence of the failure of a system includes such examples as:

- deteriorating clinical signs not recorded;
- signs recorded but their importance not understood;
- signs recorded and understood but not reported;
- signs reported but not acted upon with necessary haste;
- acted on with sufficient haste but by insufficiently experienced personnel.

It is worth considering which of the examples above are the responsibility of the nurse looking after the patient. The first four examples are the nurse's direct responsibility, not that of the attending medical staff. It is certainly possible for the nurse to influence, if not ensure that expert help of the required seniority is summoned to the deteriorating patient.

Early warning systems are now being routinely used in hospital settings to more rigorously monitor high-risk patients to recognise signs of deterioration and to increase speed of response from expert help, with the aim of preventing unnecessary cardiac arrests occurring (see Chapter 3).

REVIEW OF LEARNING
❏ The Chain of Survival has four components which are:
  - early access;
  - early recognition;
  - early defibrillation;
  - early ALS.
❏ The aim is to link essential interventions with optimising survival.

❏ Early access stresses the importance of summoning help as the first priority.
❏ Early CPR 'buys time' prior to the arrival of ALS.
❏ Early defibrillation is the most important advanced intervention.
❏ Early ALS has the aims of restoring spontaneous circulation and stabilising the casualty post-arrest.
❏ There are certain circumstances where the lone rescuer should perform CPR before telephoning for help.
❏ Out-of-hospital settings have dramatically improved access to defibrillation.
❏ The aim of a potential fifth link in the Chain of Survival is cardiac arrest prevention.
❏ In the out-of-hospital setting, the priority is to improve early recognition of and response to acute myocardial infarction.
❏ In hospital, the emphasis is on recognising patients at risk and responding quickly and effectively to prevent cardiac arrests occurring.

CONCLUSION

The Chain of Survival concept has always sought to promote the importance of reacting with speed to a cardiac arrest. The essential components rely on one another. If a single link is broken, the chain ceases to function. Today, there is greater emphasis on the prevention of cardiac arrest because it has been so difficult to significantly improve cardiac arrest survival.

REFERENCES

Ambury, P., King, B. & Bannerjee, M. (2000) Does concurrent or previous illness accurately predict cardiac arrest survival? *Resuscitation* **47**, 267–71.

Colquhoun, M.C. (2002) Defibrillation by general practitioners. *Resuscitation* **52**, 143–8.

Cummins, R., Ornato, J., Thies, W. & Pepe, P. (1991) Improving survival from cardiac arrest: the chain of survival concept. *Circulation* **83**, 1832–47.

Cummins, R.O., Eisenberg, M.S., Hallstrom, A.P. & Litwin, P.E. (1985) Survival from out-of-hospital cardiac arrest with early initiation of cardiopulmonary resuscitation. *American Journal of Emergency Medicine* **3**, 114–19.

Davies, C.S. (2002) Defibrillators in public places: the introduction of a national scheme for public access defibrillation in England. *Resuscitation* **52**, 13–21.

Department of Health (1998) *Why Mothers Die. Report of Confidential Enquiries into Maternal Deaths in the United Kingdom 1994–1996.* Department of Health, London.

Dowie, R., Campbell, H., Donohoe, R. & Clarke, P. (2003) 'Event tree' analysis of out of hospital cardiac arrest data: confirming the importance of bystander CPR. *Resuscitation* **56**, 173–81.

Eisenberg, M.S. & Mengert, T.J. (2001) Cardiac resuscitation. *New England Journal of Medicine* **344** (17), 1304–13.

Gwinnutt, C.L., Columb, M. & Harris, R. (2000) Outcome after cardiac arrest in hospitals: effect of 1997 guidelines. *Resuscitation* **47**, 125–35.

Larsen, M.P., Eisenberg, M.S., Cummins, R.O. & Hallstrom, A.P. (1993) Predicting survival from out-of-hospital cardiac arrest: a graphic model. *Annals of Emergency Medicine* **22**, 1652–8.

Mitchell, R.G., Guly, U.M., Rainer, T.H. & Robertson, C.E. (2000) Paramedic activities, drug administration and survival from out-of-hospital cardiac arrest. *Resuscitation* **43**, 95–100.

Newman, M. (1989) Chain of survival concept takes hold. *Journal of Emergency Medical Services* **14** (8), 11–13.

Newman, M. (1998) Chain of survival revisited. *Journal of Emergency Medical Services* **23** (5), 47–56.

Page, R.L., Joglar, J.A. & Kowal, R.C. (2000) Use of advisory external defibrillators by a United States airline. *New England Journal of Medicine* **343**, 1210–16.

Resuscitation Council UK (2000) *Advanced Life Support Course Provider Manual*, 4th edn. Resuscitation Council UK, London.

Valenzuela, T.D., Roe, D., Nichol, G., Clark, L.L., Spaite, D.W. & Hardman, R.G. (2000) Outcome of rapid defibrillation by security officers after cardiac arrest in casinos. *New England Journal of Medicine* **343**, 1242–7.

Young, K.D. & Siedel, J.S. (1999) Paediatric cardiopulmonary resuscitation – a collective review. *Annals of Emergency Medicine* **33**, 195–205.

Section 3

Adult Basic Life Support

6 | Adult Basic Life Support Algorithm

Pam Moule

INTRODUCTION

Adult basic life support (BLS) is employed in cardiorespiratory arrest and includes assessment of the collapsed person, maintaining airway patency, delivering expired air ventilation and external chest compressions without the aid of any equipment other than protective devices (European Resuscitation Council 2005). BLS acts to support ventilation and circulation until the causes of cardiac arrest can be ascertained and, where possible, treated with defibrillation and drugs. Any delay in the administration of such life-preserving actions can result in permanent cerebral damage and therefore BLS must be initiated, following the recommended sequence of actions, as soon as a cardiac arrest is confirmed.

AIMS

This chapter presents the principles of BLS for the layperson, in-hospital cardiac arrest for healthcare professionals and the use of automated external defibrillation (AED) in BLS.

LEARNING OUTCOMES

At the end of the chapter, the reader will be able to:

❏ identify the *safety issues* associated with BLS;
❏ describe the *sequence of actions* undertaken in BLS;
❏ describe the *techniques* of BLS delivery;
❏ understand the approach taken in *in-hospital BLS*;
❏ discuss the *management of choking adults*;
❏ describe the sequence of actions undertaken in *using the recovery position*;
❏ describe the *sequence of actions* undertaken in BLS with AED use;
❏ outline the recommendations and developments in the *use of the automated external defibrillators* in BLS.

ADULT BLS GUIDELINES

Updated resuscitation guidelines published in 2005 were based on the 'best evidence' base at the time and will no doubt continue to evolve as the availability of research knowledge in the field increases (European Resuscitation Council 2005 and International Liaison Committee on Resuscitation (ILCOR) 2005). The guidelines sought to develop a more streamlined approach to resuscitation, which differentiates between the healthcare professional, often resuscitating in the hospital environment, and the out-of-hospital rescue.

SAFETY: REDUCING RISKS IN RESUSCITATION

Prior to entering the scene of a possible cardiac arrest, the rescuer should consider the following.

- Environment – the rescuer should review all possible hazards which in an out-of-hospital arrest might present as falling debris, traffic, electricity or water. In the hospital, environmental hazards can include fluid spillage and equipment.
- Infection – the possible transmission of infection from a casualty or patient must be considered. There are only a small number of reported cases of infections such as tuberculosis (TB) and severe acute respiratory distress syndrome (SARS) being transmitted during cardiopulmonary resuscitation (CPR) and the transmission of HIV during CPR has never been reported (Handley *et al.* 2006). It is recommended that rescuers should take appropriate safety precautions in delivery of mouth-to-mouth breathing, using available protective devices, especially if the casualty is known to suffer from a serious infection such as TB (Handley *et al.* 2006).
- Manual handling – safe handling techniques should be practiced at all times, ensuring good posture during BLS and safe handling of the casualty (Resuscitation Council UK 2001).

ADULT BLS

In adult BLS, the casualty is often attended without the aid of any resuscitation equipment, such as airway adjuncts. Following assessment of safety the suggested algorithm includes responsiveness, airway and breathing. If not breathing normally, the rescuer should call for help and then proceed to call for emergency help and commence chest compressions (see Figure 6.1).

Checking for responsiveness

In the collapsed casualty, this requires a gentle shake of the casualty's shoulders whilst shouting into each ear, 'Are you all right?'

If the casualty responds verbally or by moving:

- leave the casualty where he or she is, provided this is a safe environment;
- keep checking the casualty for a verbal response or movement;
- try to establish the cause of collapse;
- ensure dignity is maintained.

If the casualty does not respond:

- shout for immediate assistance;
- continue with your assessment, which might require moving the casualty on to his or her back to gain access to the airway and pulse.

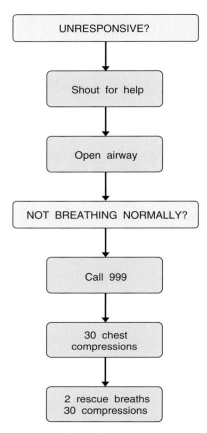

Figure 6.1 Adult basic life support algorithm. (Reproduced with kind permission from the Resuscitation Council UK.)

Opening and clearing the airway

This manoeuvre reduces the risk of airway obstruction in the unconscious or unresponsive casualty. The procedure allows lifting of the jaw, moving the tongue away from the throat.

Head tilt/chin lift
- Open the casualty's airway with a head tilt/chin lift (see Figure 6.2).
- Place one of your hands on the casualty's forehead.
- Remove any visible debris from the mouth with your finger, but leave well-fitting dentures in place.
- With the tips of the index and middle fingers of your other hand on the hard palate (the bony prominence of the chin), lift the chin to open the airway.
- In suspected cervical spine injuries, care must be taken when opening the airway, with the jaw thrust being preferred.

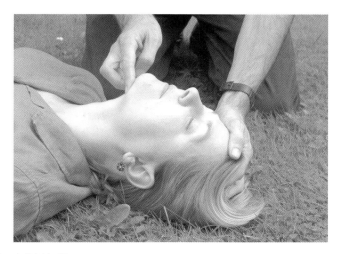

Figure 6.2 Head tilt/chin lift.

Jaw thrust (see Figure 6.3)

- This procedure is not recommended for the lay rescuer, who should employ the head tilt/chin lift procedure (see Figure 6.2).
- Some healthcare professionals may undertake the skill following training.

Look, listen and feel for breathing

Bringing the side of your face above that of the casualty, you should:

- look for signs of chest movement;
- listen for breath sounds;
- feel for breath on the side of your face.

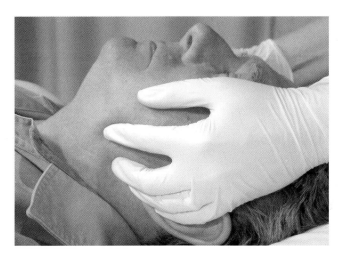

Figure 6.3 Jaw thrust.

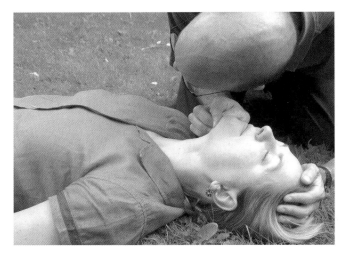

Figure 6.4 Look, listen and feel for breathing.

This manoeuvre should be completed in no more than 10 seconds (see Figure 6.4).

If the casualty is breathing normally:

- employ the recovery position (see page 70 for a fuller explanation of this);
- continue to check for breathing signs, using the look, listen and feel manoeuvre;
- send someone else to summon help if you can, and ask them to report back to you;
- if alone, leave the casualty to summon help and return to the casualty as quickly as possible.

If the casualty is not breathing normally and breath is absent or severely impaired with only occasional gasps seen:

- send someone else to call for emergency help if you can, and ask them to report back to you;
- if alone, leave the casualty to call for emergency help and return as quickly as possible to start chest compressions.

Chest compressions

The delivery of chest compressions is not delayed by an assessment for the presence of a pulse. Laypersons and healthcare professionals have difficulty making an accurate assessment of the presence or absence of the carotid pulse (Albarran *et al.* 2006, Bahr *et al.* 1997, Monsieurs *et al.* 1996). Healthcare professionals should have been taught to check for the carotid pulse (see Box 6.1):

- kneel at the side of the casualty;
- place the heel of one hand on the centre of the chest (see Figure 6.5);
- place the heel of our other hand on top;

Box 6.1   Carotid pulse check.

- Assess the carotid pulse if trained to do so.
- Maintain head tilt/chin lift throughout the procedure.
- Using the index and middle finger of your free hand, trace down the trachea of the casualty and slide across to one side to palpate the pulse between the trachea and sternocleidomastoid muscle at the side of the neck.
- Apply gentle pressure over the carotid pulse for up to 10 seconds.

- interlock the fingers of both hands to avoid compression of the ribs;
- you should ensure your own safe positioning, with knees apart, shoulders above the point of compression and elbows straight;
- compressions must be delivered with an even movement, between 4 and 5 cm in depth;
- release the chest, allowing it to rise, whilst maintaining hand contact and positioning over the point of compression;
- repeat chest compressions at the rate of 100 compressions/min until 30 have been delivered.

Rescue breathing and compressions
Combine chest compressions with rescue breaths.

Mouth-to-mouth breathing
- Open the airway again using head tilt/chin lift manoeuvre (see Figure 6.2);
- The nose should be occluded by pinching the nostrils between the index finger and thumb of the hand you have on the casualty's forehead;
- The mouth must be open whilst a head tilt/chin lift is maintained;
- You should take a deep breath and place your mouth over the casualty's mouth, ensuring a good seal
- Exhale over 1 second;
- You need to observe the chest rise and fall, which gives a measure of the effectiveness of rescue breathing;
- A further deep breath should be taken and a second breath delivered;
- If rescue breathing is not effective, try repositioning the head tilt/chin lift and check for obstructions in the casualty's mouth;
- Once two breaths have been delivered immediately re-commence chest compressions at a ratio of 30:2.

Maintain 30:2 cycle
- Cycles should not be interrupted unless the casualty starts normal breathing or shows signs of life.
- Efforts must be continued until either the casualty starts normal breathing, emergency help arrives or you are unable to maintain them.
- If there are two rescuers present then you should alternate, giving each other a break after 1 or 2 minutes to reduce fatigue.

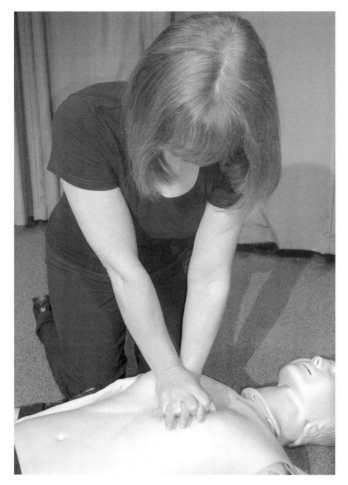

Figure 6.5 Chest compression.

Chest compression only BLS

If you are unwilling or unable to perform mouth-to-mouth breathing:

- deliver chest compressions at a continuous rate of 100 per minute without stopping;
- do not interrupt BLS unless the casualty starts normal breathing;
- continue until emergency help arrives or you are unable to continue.

Breathing

Use of mouth barriers/airway adjuncts

Rescuers may have access to barrier devices, such as face-shields or airway adjuncts. The use of face-shields is recommended, especially when attempting resuscitation in unfamiliar environments, away from home (European

Resuscitation Council 2005). The dearth of research reviewing the effectiveness of face-shields results in a lack of evidence to support their use by healthcare professionals, for whom the use of masks is recommended when available (Simmons *et al.* 1995).

Use of a mouth mask

- The mask should be placed on the casualty's face, following the manufacturer's instructions;
- The seal of the mask on the face should be ensured by placing your thumbs and fingers around the lower portion of the mask and jaw (as in Chapter 9);
- Slow breaths are delivered through the mask non-return valve;
- Chest movements should be observed.

USE OF AN AUTOMATED EXTERNAL DEFIBRILLATOR

The introduction of modern AEDs has overcome many of the obstacles associated with using manual defibrillators. Their ease of operation and safety features have meant that a broad range of first responders and rescuers are able to defibrillate without delay. Additionally, as the AED is programmed to assess the rhythm, the operator is not required to recognise or interpret cardiac arrhythmias. Due to these facilities, airline staff, paramedics and lay people with minimal training have been observed operating an AED promptly and efficiently (Capucci *et al.* 2002, Eames *et al.* 2003, Gottschalk *et al.* 2002, Page *et al.* 2000, Ross *et al.* 2001). Consequently, the European Resuscitation Council guidelines for the use of an AED have been produced (see Figure 6.6).

Chapter 11 provides further information on the use of manual defibrillators and AEDs and defibrillation. The following principles should be followed when operating an AED:

- Ensure safety of the casualty and yourself;
- Assess the casualty to establish that he or she is unresponsive and not breathing normally;
- If alone, call the emergency services and fetch the AED if available. If there is someone with you send him or her to do this;
- Commence BLS as soon as possible, delivering 30 chest compressions and two breaths (see Chest compressions section);
- When the defibrillator arrives:
  - switch on the AED
  - attach the adhesive electrodes in the correct position and connect the cable to the patient (see Figures 6.7(a)–6.7(c))
  - if more than one rescuer is present, BLS should continue
  - follow the directions (visual and spoken)
  - ensure no one is touching the patient during rhythm analysis
- If shock advised (see Figures 6.8(a)–6.8(b)):
  - ensure no one is in contact with the casualty; shout, 'stand clear, every one clear' and confirm bystander and operator safety

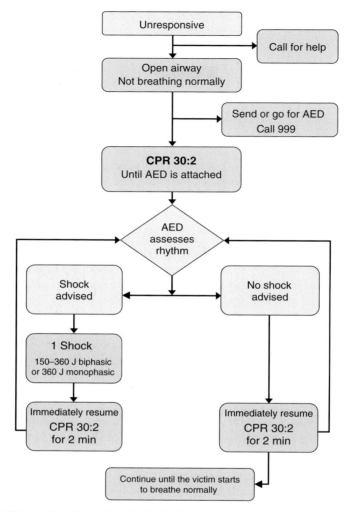

Figure 6.6 AED algorithm. (Reproduced with kind permission from the Resuscitation Council UK.)

- ○ shout, 'shocking casualty' and press the shock button as directed by the AED (Fully automated AEDs will deliver the shock without your intervention.)
- ○ continue as directed by the voice prompts
- If no shock advised:
  - ○ resume BLS at a ratio of 30 compressions and 2 rescue breaths
  - ○ continue as advised by the voice or visual prompts until either:
    - – qualified help arrives
    - – the casualty recommences normal breathing
    - – you are too tired to continue.

It is important that any rescuers or bystanders do not touch the casualty during the analysis of heart rhythm as this may lead to artifactual errors that can lead

(a)

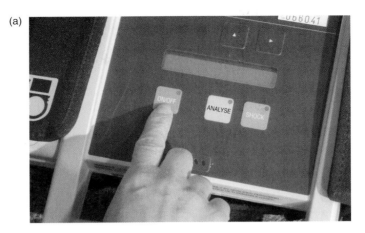

(b)

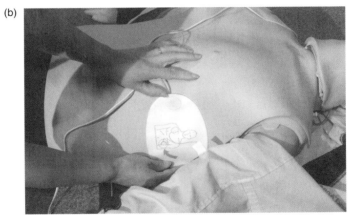

(c)

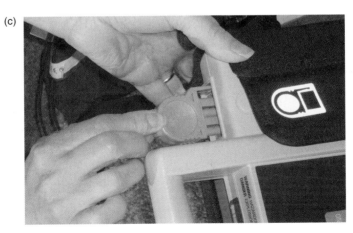

Figure 6.7 (a) Switching on AED. (b) Positioning of electrodes. (c) Connecting electrodes to AED.

(a)

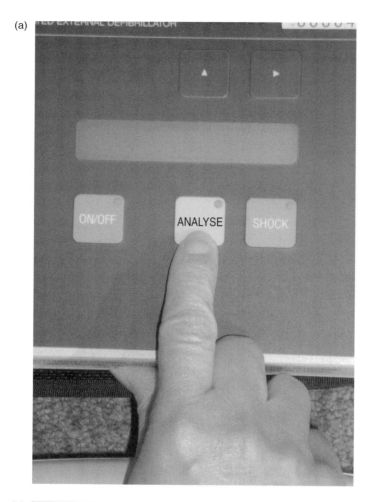

(b)

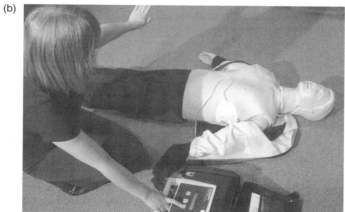

Figure 6.8 (a) Analysis of rhythm. (b) Preparing to defibrillate.

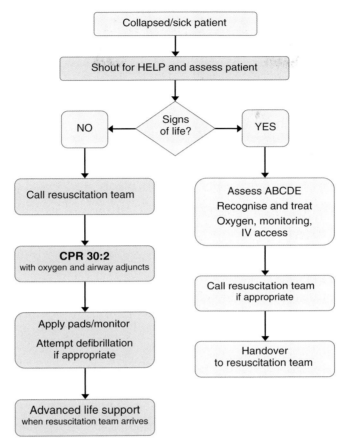

Figure 6.9 In-hospital resuscitation algorithm. (Reproduced with kind permission from the Resuscitation Council UK.)

to unwanted delays. The defibrillator may interpret abnormal heart rhythms of ventricular fibrillation (VF) or ventricular tachycardia (VT) as artifact.

AEDs vary in the level of sophistication. In some fully automatic models, the machine will automatically analyse heart rhythm and having detected a shockable rhythm will deliver a shock without further need for input. This reduces the risk of rescuer error and delays.

IN-HOSPITAL RESUSCITATION

This approach is emphasised for use by healthcare professionals attending the collapsed patient in the hospital setting. The provision of resuscitation equipment within the hospital and some pre-hospital settings, such as ambulance paramedics, necessitates the modification of BLS guidelines. The initial management of cardiac arrest in these circumstances is depicted in the in-hospital resuscitation algorithm (see Figure 6.9). For further information on the management of advanced life support (ALS) in hospital, see Chapter 7.

Patient collapse

Once safety of the environment is established, the healthcare professional should call for help and check for patient response. Once colleagues are available to help, a number of actions can be undertaken in the initial phase of managing a cardiac arrest.

If the patient responds:

- summon the local medical emergency team;
- assess the patient using ABCDE (see Chapter 3);
- start to administer oxygen;
- attach ECG monitoring leads and commence monitoring;
- secure venous access if this is not already in place.

If there is no response from the patient:

- shout for help unless present;
- ensure the patient is lying prone and open the airway with head tilt/chin lift (see Figure 6.2);
- look, listen and feel for breathing for up to 10 seconds (see Figure 6.4);
- look for obstructions in the mouth and remove obvious debris;
- those with clinical assessment skills may assess the carotid pulse for up to 10 seconds, either simultaneously or following breathing checks.

If the patient has a pulse and/or signs of life are present:

- summon the local medical emergency team;
- assess the patient using ABCDE (see Chapter 3);
- administer oxygen (see Chapter 9);
- commence cardiac monitoring (see Chapter 10);
- obtain venous access (see Chapter 12).

If the patient has no pulse or signs of life:

- commence CPR using oxygen and airway adjuncts;
- ensure resuscitation equipment and the defibrillator are accessible at the patient's side;
- support the airway and ventilation using available equipment, such as a pocket mask, oropharyngeal airway, LMA or bag-valve-mask (see Chapter 4 for further explanation of this equipment);
- ensure oxygen is delivered;
- proceed in delivering 30 chest compressions followed by two ventilations, until the patient is intubated with a secure cuffed tracheal tube or LMA;
- as a priority, the electrodes of either a manual or AED should be attached to the patient and used as necessary (see Chapter 11 for further explanation);
- intravenous access should be secured, if not already available;
- you should prepare to hand over to the arriving medical emergency team, providing access to the patient's notes;
- if the patient's relatives or other patients are in the vicinity, ensure members of the team are available to provide appropriate support.

Respiratory arrest
If on assessment, the patient is not breathing but has a pulse, give oxygen. Check the pulse after every ten breaths or minute.

Witnessed and monitored cardiac arrest
- Assess patient ABCDE and confirm cardiac arrest;
- Call for local help and contact the medical emergency team;
- If the patient is in confirmed VT/VF and a defibrillator is not available, administer a pre-cordial thump only if trained to do so;
- If patient is in confirmed VT/VF and a defibrillator is available, apply pads/manual paddles and deliver one shock;
- Continue ALS (see Chapter 7).

Recovery position
There is no one recovery position, though the placement of an unconscious casualty in a lateral position with no pressure on the chest is vital in maintaining support of the airway, as it ensures the tongue is held in a forward position and it reduces the chance of inhalation of any expelled gastric contents (European Resuscitation Council 2005).

Whilst placing someone in the recovery position, make sure you maintain your own good posture and prevent injuries to yourself and the casualty.

- Make sure the environment is safe; check for potential hazards such as broken glass.
- Remove any hazards from the casualty, such as work tools or spectacles.
- Kneel next to the casualty.
- Ensure the casualty has straight legs and is lying on his or her back.
- Move the arm closest to you so that it is at right angles to the casualty's body, with the palm of the hand facing upwards.
- The other arm should be positioned across the chest, with the back of the hand placed next to the casualty's cheek. The hand should be held in this position.
- The leg furthest away from you should be bent at the knee, ensuring the foot is in contact with the ground.
- Pull on the leg, whilst maintaining hold of the hand on the cheek, to roll the casualty towards you onto his or her side.
- Move the upper leg to ensure it is at right angles to the casualty, supporting a stable position.
- Ensure the airway is open, tilting the head back if necessary and using the hand to support the positioning of the head (see Figures 6.10(a)–6.10(d) and Box 6.2).

Box 6.2   Best practice – monitoring the casualty in the recovery position.

Frequently check breathing rate and depth.

Observe the circulation to the lower arm that the casualty is lying on.

Turn the casualty onto his or her opposite side if he or she is required to remain in the recovery position for more than 30 minutes.

Preserve dignity throughout.

(a)

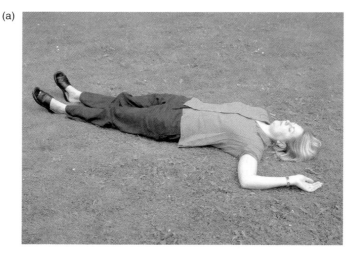

(b)

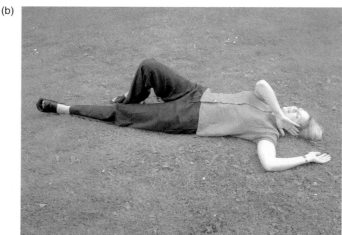

Figure 6.10 (a) Putting the patient in the recovery position. (b) Putting the patient in the recovery position.

Choking foreign body airway obstruction

Choking is commonly associated with the intake of food and can therefore be witnessed, allowing early response. Foreign bodies can lead to mild or severe airway obstruction.

The choking algorithm (see Figure 6.11) suggests that there should be an initial assessment of the casualty, when you ask 'Are you choking?'

If the casualty is clutching his or her throat, able to speak and answer your question, cough and breathe, he or she is suffering from mild airway obstruction. If the casualty is unable to speak, unable to breathe or is wheezing and is unable to cough, he or she has a severe airway obstruction and may be unconscious or lapse into unconsciousness.

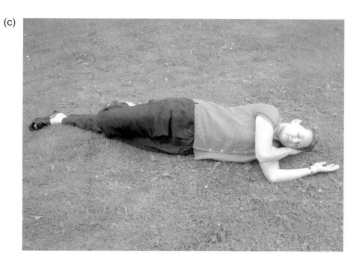

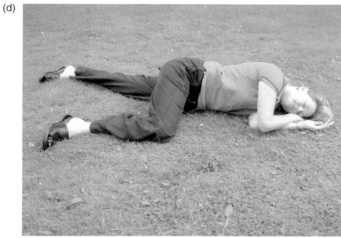

Figure 6.10 (c) Putting the patient in the recovery position. (d) The recovery position.

Mild airway obstruction

If the casualty appears to be choking but is conscious and coughing, no further action should be necessary other than to encourage continued coughing, observing for relief of the obstruction.

Severe airway obstruction – casualty conscious

Perform the following manoeuvres.

- Deliver five back blows. Stand to the side and slightly behind the casualty. Encourage the casualty to lean forwards, to support outward projection of any obstruction. Deliver up to five blows with the heel of your hand, between the scapulae (see Figure 6.12);
- Check to see if the obstruction is relieved;

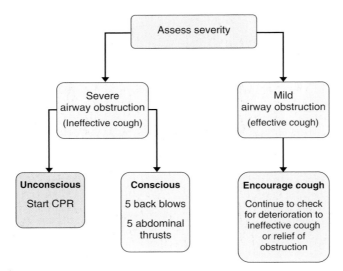

Figure 6.11 Choking algorithm. (Reproduced with kind permission from the Resuscitation Council UK.)

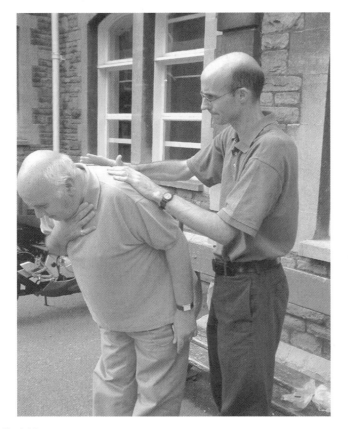

Figure 6.12 Back blows.

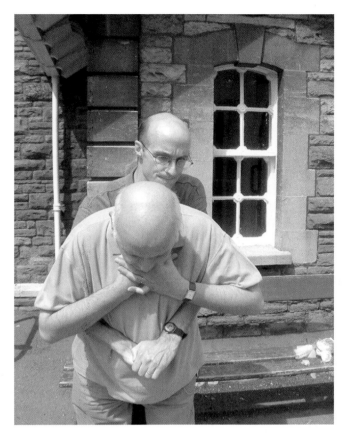

Figure 6.13 Abdominal thrusts.

- If the obstruction persists, deliver up to five abdominal thrusts. Stand behind the casualty, wrap your arms around the waist and ensure the casualty is leaning forwards. Make a fist with one hand and close the other hand on top of it. Position your hands below the xiphisternum. Pull your hands inwards and upwards (see Figure 6.13). Check to see if the obstruction has cleared;
- Up to five back blows and five abdominal thrusts can be alternated until the obstruction is cleared;
- If the casualty becomes unconscious, undertake the following procedures.

Severe airway obstruction – casualty unconscious

If back blows and abdominal thrusts fail and the casualty becomes unconscious, a sequence of life support is recommended, as in the managing of the choking adult algorithm (European Resuscitation Council 2005) (see Figure 6.11).

- Ensure safe positioning of the casualty on the ground;
- Call Emergency Medical Team;

- Commence BLS with 30 chest compressions (recommended even if the pulse is present (Handley *et al.* 2006), followed by delivery of two breaths as specified above under chest compressions;
- The casualty may require medical assessment and treatment following these interventions.

REVIEW OF LEARNING

❏ BLS includes assessing safety of the environment, checking response, opening and clearing the airway, checking breathing, delivering chest compressions, if required, and combined chest compressions and breathing if needed (30:2).

❏ It is important to call for emergency help after establishing the presence or absence of breathing.

❏ It is important to commence BLS without delay with 30 chest compressions followed by two rescue breaths.

❏ If an AED is available, immediate defibrillation should be given.

❏ In-hospital resuscitation is emphasised for use by healthcare personnel.

❏ The recovery position is vital in maintaining the support of the airway in the collapsed casualty.

❏ The management of foreign body airway obstruction depends on its severity.

Case study

Mr Coughlin, a 73-year-old, is visiting his son in his new home. He has been digging the garden and comes into the house clutching his chest. He collapses to the floor and his wife and son are unable to rouse him. The son rushes across the street to find help. You are one of two rescuers who attend the house. You are both student nurses who have recently had BLS training.

What should you do?

Before reading on, make a list of your actions.

Firstly, you should check that the environment is safe to enter, then assess the casualty for a response. Next, you should open and clear the airway and check for the presence of breathing. This reveals that Mr Coughlin is unresponsive and not breathing. Your friend goes to contact the emergency services. There are no signs of life and on checking the pulse, you find this is also absent. After phoning for help, your friend explains to Mr Coughlin's wife and son about the need to perform BLS.

In line with guidelines, you commence BLS. You deliver 30 chest compressions followed by two ventilations for 2 minutes before your friend takes over.

After 20 minutes, the emergency services arrive and are able to apply defibrillator pads and administer oxygen via a mask, whilst you continue BLS. This unfortunately reveals that Mr Coughlin has no cardiac output and an asystolic rhythm is seen on the monitor screen.

CONCLUSION

The guidelines for BLS are designed to aid recall and support effective resuscitation and all healthcare professionals should be familiar with the most up-to-date guidelines. Accessing the *Resuscitation* journal and Resuscitation Council UK and European Resuscitation Council websites (www.resus.org.uk and www.erc.edu) will ensure that practice remains updated.

REFERENCES

Albarran, J., Moule, P., Soar, J. & Gilchrist, M. (2006) A comparison of simultaneous and sequential checking of breathing and pulse by healthcare providers. *Resuscitation* **68** (2), 243–9.

Bahr, J., Klinger, H., Panzer W., Rode, H. & Kettler, D. (1997) Skills of lay people checking the carotid pulse. *Resuscitation* **35**, 23–6.

Capucci, A., Ascheri, D., Pieploi, M., Bardy, G., Iconomu, E. & Arverdi, M. (2002) Tripling survival from sudden cardiac arrest via early defibrillation without traditional education in cardiopulmonary resuscitation. *Circulation* **106**, 1065–70.

Eames, P., Larsen, P. & Galletly, D. (2003) Comparison of ease of use of three automated defibrillators by untrained people. *Resuscitation* **58**, 25–30.

European Resuscitation Council (2005) European Resuscitation Council guidelines for resuscitation 2005. *Resuscitation* **67** (suppl 1), S7–23, S25–37.

Gottschalk, A., Burmeister, M., Freitag, M., Cavus, E. & Standl, T. (2002) Influence of early defibrillation on the survival rate and quality of life after CPR in prehospital emergency medical service in a German metropolitan area. *Resuscitation* **53**, 15–20.

Handley, A., Koster, R., Monsieurs, K., Perkins, G., Davies, S. & Bossaert, L. (2006) Adult basic life support and use of automated external defibrillators. In: Baskett, P. & Nolan, M. (eds) *A Pocket Book of the European Resuscitation Council Guidelines for Resuscitation 2005*. Mosby Elsevier, Edinburgh, pp. 8–13.

International Liaison Committee on Resuscitation (2005) International consensus on cardiopulmonary resuscitation and emergency cardiovascular care science with treatment recommendations. *Resuscitation* **67**, 187–211.

Monsieurs, K., De Cauwer, H. & Bossaert, L. (1996) Feeling for carotid pulse: is five seconds enough? *Resuscitation* **31**, S3.

Page, J., Kowol, R. & Zagrodsky, J. (2000) The use of automated external defibrillators by US airline. *New England Journal of Medicine* **343** (17), 1210–16.

Resuscitation Council UK (2001) *Guidance on Safe Handling*. Resuscitation Council UK, London. Available online at: http://www.resus.org.uk/pages/safehand.pdf.

Ross, P., Nolan, J., Hill, E., Dawson, J., Whimser, F. & Skinner, D. (2001) The use of AEDs by police officers in the city of London. *Resuscitation* **50**, 141–6.

Simmons, M., Deano, D., Moon, L., Peters, K. & Cavanaugh, S. (1995) Bench evaluation: three face shield CPR barrier devices. *Respiratory Care* **40**, 618–23.

Websites

Resuscitation Council UK – www.resus.org.uk
European Resuscitation Council – www.erc.edu

Section 4

Advanced Life Support

The Advanced Life Support Algorithm

Jackie Younker

INTRODUCTION

Advanced life support (ALS) is an essential link in the Chain of Survival. The algorithm provides a sequence of actions for the management of all people who appear in cardiac arrest – unconscious, unresponsive and without signs of life. Cardiac arrest may present as a *shockable* rhythm, such as ventricular fibrillation or pulseless ventricular tachycardia (VF/VT), or a *non-shockable* rhythm, such as asystole or pulseless electrical activity (PEA). Attempts at defibrillation will be necessary in cases of VF/VT. Other actions, including chest compressions, airway management and ventilation, venous access, drug administration and correction of possible causes, are common to both these rhythms. The algorithm is applicable universally but cardiac arrest may occur in special circumstances, for example anaphylaxis, asthma and drug overdose. Additional interventions may be necessary, as discussed in Chapter 15.

During ALS, the focus must be on early defibrillation and high-quality uninterrupted cardiopulmonary resuscitation (CPR). The ALS algorithm was based on collaborative research from resuscitation experts around the world. All information in this chapter is drawn from the references noted at the end.

AIMS

This chapter expands on each step of the ALS treatment algorithm (see Figure 7.1).

LEARNING OUTCOMES

At the end of the chapter, the reader will be able to:

❑ describe the *sequence of actions* in the ALS algorithm;
❑ understand the management of *patients in a shockable rhythm* (VF/VT);
❑ understand the management of *patients in a non-shockable rhythm* (PEA and asystole).

SHOCKABLE RHYTHMS: VF/VT

The majority of people who collapse from a cardiac arrest in the community are in VF and those who are most likely to survive (ILCOR 2005a). Whatever

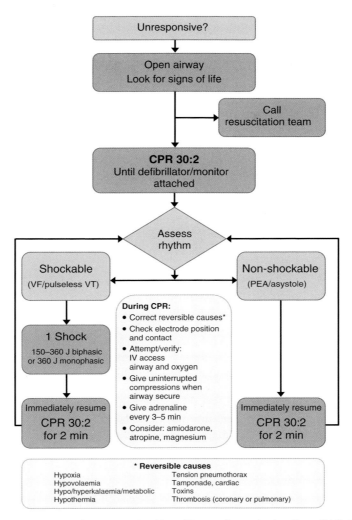

Figure 7.1 Adult advanced life support algorithm. (*Source*: Resuscitation Council UK, Resuscitation Guidelines 2005. Reproduced with kind permission of the Resuscitation Council UK.)

the setting, hospital, community or home, successful resuscitation depends on early defibrillation (Deakin & Nolan 2005). The chance of successful defibrillation declines with each minute that VF persists. While effective basic life support (BLS) slows the irreversible damage, it cannot stop it. The patient's rhythm needs to be assessed as soon as possible with monitoring electrodes from an automatic or manual defibrillator. The first shock should be delivered as soon as possible if the rhythm is VF/VT (for further information about these arrhythmias, see Chapter 10). If a monitor is not available, CPR should be continued until a defibrillator arrives.

The following provides a step-by-step account of treatment of *shockable* rhythms (VF/VT) according to the ALS algorithm (see Figure 7.1).

Chest compressions

CPR should be started after confirming cardiac arrest with chest compressions at a ratio of 30:2, as described in Chapter 6. It is important not to delay the starting of chest compressions and continue until a defibrillator is available.

Treating *shockable* rhythms (VF/VT)

- Attempt defibrillation – give one shock of 150–200 J biphasic (360 J monophasic);
- Immediately resume chest compressions (30:2) without checking the rhythm or feeling for a pulse. The time between shock delivery and beginning with chest compressions should not exceed 10 seconds. Giving chest compressions even in the presence of a perfusing rhythm does not increase the chance of VF recurring and is not harmful to the patient (Nolan *et al.* 2005);
- Continue CPR for 2 minutes, then pause compressions briefly to check the monitor.

Persistent VF/VT

- Give a second shock of 150–200 J biphasic (360 J monophasic);
- Resume CPR immediately and continue for 2 minutes;
- Pause compressions briefly to check the monitor;
- If VF/VT persists – administer adrenaline 1 mg IV, then immediately follow with a third shock of 150–200 J biphasic (360 J monophasic). The adrenaline should be ready to give, so the delay between stopping chest compressions and giving a shock is minimised. If the adrenaline is not ready, give it after the shock rather than delaying the shock;
- Resume CPR immediately and continue for 2 minutes;
- If VF/VT persists – administer amiodarone 300 mg IV, then immediately follow with a fourth shock of 150–200 J biphasic (360 J monophasic);
- Resume CPR immediately and continue for 2 minutes;
- Give adrenaline 1 mg IV immediately before alternate shocks. This is approximately every 3–5 minutes;
- Give further shocks after each 2-minute period of CPR if VF/VT persists on the monitor;
- Poor electrode or paddle contact will reduce the chances of successful defibrillation (Bradbury *et al.* 2000). A number of factors can impact on the effectiveness of defibrillation including position of the paddles or pads, for example consider anteroposterior (refer to Chapter 11).

Rhythm changes

Organised electrical activity compatible with a pulse may be seen on the monitor during the brief pause after 2 minutes of chest compressions. If present, check for a pulse. If a pulse is present, start post-resuscitation care. An organised rhythm may be noted on the monitor before completion of 2 minutes for CPR. Chest compressions should not be stopped unless the patient shows signs of life indicating a return of spontaneous circulation (Resuscitation Council UK 2006). If no pulse is present, continue CPR and begin treating the patient according to the non-shockable side of the algorithm.

If asystole is seen on the monitor during the brief pause, continue CPR and begin treating the patient according to the non-shockable side of the algorithm.

It may be difficult to distinguish between very fine VF and asystole. If there is any doubt, do not attempt defibrillation. Chest compressions and ventilation should be continued.

Precordial thump

- A single precordial thump is an acceptable and possibly helpful action in a witnessed or monitored VF/VT arrest when a defibrillator is not immediately available (ILCOR 2005a).
- Give a sharp blow with a closed fist on the patient's sternum. If this is done quickly after the cardiac arrest, it may be enough to successfully convert the patient's heart back to a perfusing rhythm. Precordial thump should be given only by healthcare professionals trained in the technique.
- Reassess circulation after delivery of a precordial thump.

NON-SHOCKABLE RHYTHMS: PEA/ASYSTOLE

The outcome for 'non-shockable' rhythms is poor (ILCOR 2005b). PEA is present when organised cardiac electrical activity is present on the monitor but the pulse is not palpable. PEA and asystole may be caused by conditions that are reversible if found and treated quickly and effectively.

Treating PEA

- Start CPR 30:2;
- Give adrenaline 1 mg IV as soon as intravascular access is obtained;
- Continue CPR 30:2 until the airway is secured. Chest compressions can be continued without pausing for ventilation when an advanced airway is in place (refer to Chapter 9 for airway management);
- Pause briefly to check the rhythm after 2 minutes;
- If organised electrical activity is seen, check the patient for signs of life and/or pulse. If signs of life and/or pulse are present, begin post-resuscitation care. If no signs of life are present, persistent PEA, continue CPR;
- Pause briefly every 2 minutes to recheck the rhythm and treat the patient as appropriate;
- Further adrenaline should be given every 3–5 minutes or alternate loops of the algorithm;
- If the rhythm changes to VF/VT, change to the shockable side of the algorithm;
- If asystole is seen on the monitor, continue CPR and recheck the rhythm every 2 minutes. Give adrenaline 1 mg IV every 3–5 minutes.

Treating asystole and slow PEA (rate <60 per minute)

- Start CPR 30:2;
- Confirm that monitoring leads are attached correctly without stopping CPR;

- Give adrenaline 1 mg IV as soon as intravascular access is obtained;
- Give atropine 3 mg IV once;
- Continue CPR 30:2 until the airway is secured. Chest compressions can be continued without pausing for ventilation when an advanced airway is in place (refer to Chapter 9 for airway management);
- Pause briefly to check the rhythm after 2 minutes and treat accordingly;
- Further adrenaline should be given every 3–5 minutes or alternate loops of the algorithm;
- If the rhythm changes to VF/VT, change to the shockable side of the algorithm;
- Check the ECG carefully for the presence of a P wave or slow ventricular activity. These rhythms may respond to cardiac pacing (Deakin & Nolan 2005).

During CPR

- Chest compressions – good quality chest compressions are important during the treatment of persistent VF/VT or PEA/asystole. Providing CPR at a ratio of 30:2 is tiring. The individual doing compressions should be changed every 2 minutes to prevent fatigue and maintain the consistent quality of compressions.
- Airway and ventilation – it will be impossible to restart the heart without adequate oxygenation. Secure the patient's airway and deliver the highest possible concentration of oxygen. Tracheal intubation is the most reliable means to secure the airway, but a trained and experienced healthcare provider must perform this (Nolan *et al.* 2005). Chest compressions should not be interrupted during intubation except briefly to pass the tube through the vocal cords. Alternatively, tracheal intubation can be deferred until return of spontaneous circulation. An LMA or combitube may be inserted instead. Once the trachea has been intubated, chest compressions should be performed at a continuous rate of 100 per minute, stopping only for defibrillation or return of spontaneous circulation (Resuscitation Council 2006). Ventilation should be continued at approximately ten breaths/min. If an LMA has been inserted, attempt to perform continuous chest compressions, uninterrupted during ventilation. If this is not possible due to excessive gas leakage resulting in inadequate ventilation, use a compression-to-ventilation ratio of 30:2 (see Chapter 6).
- Intravenous access – an intravenous line is essential for giving drugs and fluids. This can be achieved by central or peripheral venous access. Central veins are ideal because drugs can be delivered rapidly into the circulation. Cannulation of a peripheral vein is the procedure of choice because it is quicker, easier and safer.
- Drugs – the drugs administered by the peripheral route must be followed by at least a 20-mL flush of 0.9% saline and, if possible, elevation of the extremity (Resuscitation Council UK 2006). Pre-filled syringes which are described in Chapter 12 may be used.
- Reversible causes – consider the potential causes or aggravating factors that can be treated specifically. These are divided into four H's and four T's to help remember them during the cardiac arrest (see Chapter 13).

REVIEW OF LEARNING

❑ The ALS algorithm provides a sequence of actions for the management of all people who appear in cardiac arrest, namely those who are unconscious, unresponsive and without signs of life.

❑ Cardiac arrest may present as a 'shockable' rhythm, such as VF/VT, or a 'non-shockable' rhythm, such as asystole or PEA.

❑ The chance of successful defibrillation declines with each minute that VF persists. The first shock should be delivered as soon as possible if the rhythm is VF/VT.

❑ The outcome for 'non-shockable' rhythms is poor. The team must rapidly consider and effectively treat the potentially reversible causes.

CONCLUSION

The ALS algorithm provides a guide for the actions to take and decisions to make for all patients who appear to be in cardiac arrest. It is divided into shockable and non-shockable rhythms. All those involved in carrying out ALS should keep abreast of the most up-to-date guidelines by regularly accessing the *Resuscitation* journal and Resuscitation Council UK and European Resuscitation Council websites (www.resus.org.uk and www.rec.edu/).

REFERENCES

Bradbury, N., Hyde, D. & Nolan, J. (2000) Reliability of ECG monitoring with a gel pad/paddle combination after defibrillation. *Resuscitation* **44**, 203–6.

Deakin, C.D. & Nolan, J.P. (2005) European Resuscitation Council guidelines for resuscitation 2005. Section 3: electrical therapies. Automated external defibrillators, defibrillation, cardioversion and pacing. *Resuscitation* **67** (suppl I), 25–37.

International Liaison Committee on Resuscitation (ILCOR) (2005a). Part 3: defibrillation. International consensus on cardiopulmonary resuscitation and emergency cardiovascular care science with treatment recommendations. *Resuscitation* **67**, 203–11.

International Liaison Committee on Resuscitation (ILCOR) (2005b). Part 4: advanced life support. International consensus on cardiopulmonary resuscitation and emergency cardiovascular care science with treatment recommendations. *Resuscitation* **67**, 213–47.

Nolan, J.P., Deakin, C.D., Soar, J., Bottiger, B.W. & Smith, G. (2005) European Resuscitation Council guidelines for resuscitation 2005. Section 4: adult advanced life support. *Resuscitation* **67** (suppl I), 39–86.

Resuscitation Council UK (2006) *Advanced Life Support Course Provider Manual*, 5th edn. Resuscitation Council UK, London.

Section 5

Paediatric Life Support

8 | Paediatric Life Support

Rebecca Hoskins

INTRODUCTION

Paediatric cardiac arrest is fortunately an infrequent event. Only 2% of all out-of-hospital cardiac arrests occur in children (Engdahl *et al.* 2003). One of the most common causes of cardiac arrest and death in children between 1 and 16 years is trauma (Donoghue *et al.* 2005). Unfortunately, the outcome of paediatric cardiac arrest is poor; the child who has suffered a respiratory arrest has a long-term survival rate of 50–70% whereas for a child in cardiorespiratory arrest, the survival rate is 5% (European Resuscitation Council (ERC) 2005). One reason identified for poor outcomes is that most paediatric cardiac arrests are respiratory in origin, with prolonged progressive anoxia preceding asystolic cardiac arrest and making recovery of major organ systems unlikely (Byrne & Phillips 2003). The differing aetiology of cardiac arrest in children and infants means that some small but important differences exist compared with the adults and these have been emphasised in the most recent resuscitation guidelines.

The International Liaison Committee on Resuscitation (ILCOR 2005) paediatric task force reviewed the current research and evidence base which underpins practice in paediatric resuscitation and made some key new recommendations. This chapter presents the current UK resuscitation paediatric guidelines (Resuscitation Council UK 2005).

AIMS

This chapter presents the principles of basic life support (BLS) and advanced life support (ALS) in infants and children.

LEARNING OUTCOMES

At the end of the chapter, the reader will be able to:

❏ describe the sequence of actions undertaken in paediatric BLS;
❏ discuss the differences in causes in cardiac arrest in children and infants;
❏ discuss the management of choking children and infants;
❏ describe the differences between paediatric and adult BLS and ALS algorithms;
❏ understand the management of shockable and non-shockable rhythms in children;

Paediatric basic life support

(Healthcare professionals
with a duty to respond)

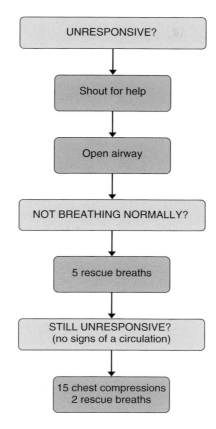

After 1 minute, call resuscitation team then continue CPR

Figure 8.1 Basic life support paediatric algorithm. (*Source*: Resuscitation Council UK, Resuscitation Guidelines 2005. Reproduced with kind permission of the Resuscitation Council UK.)

❑ discuss the intraosseous route of drug administration in children;
❑ be able to calculate appropriate drug doses.

BASIC LIFE SUPPORT IN INFANTS AND CHILDREN (see Figure 8.1)

The previous distinctions between infants, young children and older children have been simplified in the latest resuscitation guidelines. A single compression–ventilation ratio (30:2) for lay rescuers of children and adults is now recommended (ILCOR 2005). One important reason for the streamlining and simplifying of the algorithm has been to ensure that rescuers feel able to commence BLS even if they have not received specific training in paediatric resuscitation. There is good evidence to suggest that the earlier bystander life support is initiated the better the chance of survival (Berg *et al.* 2000). It is important to note that some differences in BLS still exist because of the physiological differences in children.

The Resuscitation Council UK (2005) adopts the following definitions to differentiate age groups:

- An infant is a child under the age of one year.
- A child is aged between one year and puberty.

Differences in the aetiology of cardiac arrest in children reflect the management priorities of BLS; however, a safe approach is a fundamental component of all the guidelines.

Checking for responsiveness

The next priority is to ascertain whether the child is responsive to voice or gentle stimulation. Placing a hand on the child's forehead will ensure that a potential cervical spine injury is not exacerbated. It is important not to shake an infant or a child because of the risk of cerebral injury associated with shaking. Asking the child if he or she is alright should elicit a response such as eye opening even in the pre-verbal child.

If the child responds by crying, speaking or moving:

Child should be left in the position in which he or she is found unless in immediate danger.

The condition of the child should be regularly assessed and if help is needed, this should be sought.

If the child does not respond then the rescuer should:

Shout for help:

- Open the child's airway using a head tilt and chin lift manoeuvre in the position in which the child is found (see Figures 8.2 and 8.3).

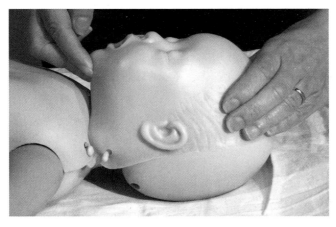

Figure 8.2 Opening airway in the infant

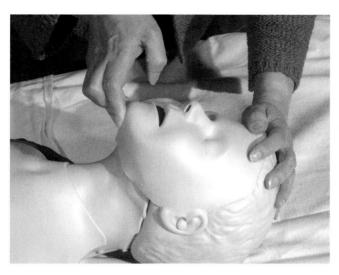

Figure 8.3 Opening the airway in the child.

- It is important not to apply pressure to the soft tissues as this can occlude the narrow airway.
- A jaw thrust manoeuvre can be carried out if a neck injury is suspected or a chin lift head tilt manoeuvre is not successful.

Then for no more than 10 seconds the rescuer should:

look for chest movements;
listen at the child's nose and mouth for breath sounds;
feel for air movement.

If the child is breathing normally:

Turn the child onto his side into the recovery position and check for continued breathing.

If the child is not breathing or is making ineffective (agonal) gasps:

- Any obvious obstruction should be removed (a blind finger sweep should not be used).
- Five initial rescue breaths should be given. The nose should be gently pinched and the breath delivered over 1–1.5 seconds. The chest should be seen to rise to confirm that ventilation breaths have been effective. This should be repeated, ensuring the rescuer takes a new breath himself or herself each time he or she delivers an expired ventilated. In infants, the nose and mouth should be covered by the rescuer's mouth.
- If the chest does not rise, the airway should be adjusted slightly (the head should be in the neutral position for an infant and 'sniffing the morning air' in a child to ensure an optimum open airway position).

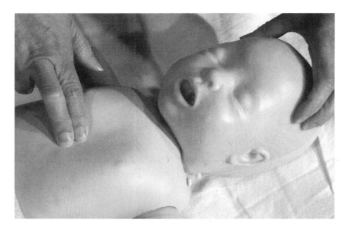

Figure 8.4   Chest compressions in the infant.

- If the chest does not move after five attempts, the rescuer should move on to chest compressions. At the same time, the child should be observed for any signs of life (movement, gag reflex and groaning).

Check for signs of a circulation:

Rescuers should take no more than 10 seconds to assess for signs of life.
Check a pulse (in an infant, the brachial pulse should be assessed; in a child, the carotid pulse can be assessed).

If the rescuer is able to feel a pulse:

Rescue breathing should be continued until the child is breathing effectively. Once the presence of breathing is confirmed, the child must be turned on his or her side if he or she remains unconscious. Assess the child at frequent intervals.
If either there are no signs of circulation or there is no pulse, or the pulse is less than 60 beats/min with poor perfusion, then chest compressions and ventilation should be commenced (Resuscitation Council UK 2005).

For infants and children, the lower third of the sternum should be depressed (one finger breadth up from the xiphisternum) (see Figures 8.4 and 8.5). Evidence now suggests that the previous recommendation in infants could result in compression over the upper abdomen (Clements & McGowan 2000). The depth of the chest compressions should depress the sternum approximately one-third the diameter of the chest. The rate of compressions should be 100 per minute and the ratio of compressions to ventilations should be:

15:2   for two or more rescuers and
30:2   for a lone rescuer.

In an infant, the lone rescuer should use two fingers to depress the sternum (see Figure 8.5); if two rescuers are available the encircling technique should be employed. This method has been found to be more effective in increasing coronary perfusion (Kinney & Tibballs 1999). In children over the age of one

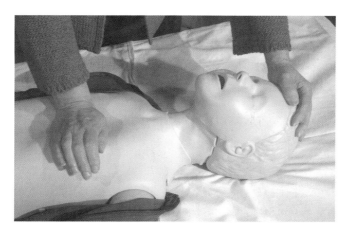

Figure 8.5 Chest compressions with one hand.

year, compressions should be delivered by the rescuer's placing the heel of one hand over the lower third of the sternum (see Figure 8.5). In larger children or for small rescuers both hands can be used to deliver the compressions and depress one-third of the depth of the child's chest (see Figure 8.6).

Compressions and ventilations should be continued until:

- the child shows signs of life;
- help arrives;
- the rescuer becomes exhausted.

Phoning for help:

If a child collapses in hospital, a cardiac arrest call should go out simultaneously while BLS measures are instituted.

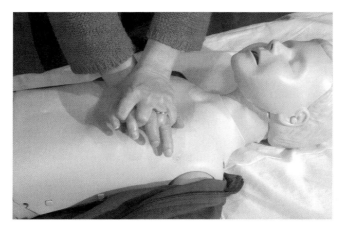

Figure 8.6 Chest compression in the larger child using two hands.

Paediatric FBAO treatment

```
                        ┌─────────────────────┐
                        │   Assess severity   │
                        └─────────────────────┘
              ┌────────────────────┐    ┌────────────────────┐
              │  Ineffective cough │    │   Effective cough  │
              └────────────────────┘    └────────────────────┘

   ┌──────────────┐  ┌──────────────┐  ┌──────────────────┐
   │ Unconscious  │  │  Conscious   │  │  Encourage cough │
   │              │  │              │  │                  │
   │ Open airway  │  │ 5 back blows │  │ Continue to check│
   │  5 breaths   │  │  5 thrusts   │  │ for deterioration│
   │  Start CPR   │  │(chest for    │  │  to ineffective  │
   │              │  │   infant)    │  │      cough       │
   │              │  │ (abdominal   │  │   or relief of   │
   │              │  │ for child >1)│  │    obstruction   │
   └──────────────┘  └──────────────┘  └──────────────────┘
```

Figure 8.7   Paediatric choking algorithm. (*Source*: Resuscitation Council UK, Resuscitation Guidelines 2005. Reproduced with kind permission of the Resuscitation Council UK.)

For out-of-hospital arrests, the decision whether to phone fast (after a minute of BLS) or to phone first is made when an assessment of the cause of the collapse has been established. In event that the sudden collapse of a child is witnessed, rescuers should phone first in order to gain early access to defibrillation as the cause of the collapse is likely to be due to an arrhythmia. However, in the majority of cases the cardiac arrest will have been preceded by a period of hypoxia which may be reversed by a minute of ventilation and compressions. If nobody is available, rescuers should go for help after a minute of BLS.

Recognition and response to foreign body airway obstruction in infants and children (see Figure 8.7)

It is important to recognise the cause of airway obstruction as quickly as possible so the appropriate management can be initiated. The majority of deaths from foreign body aspiration occur in pre-school children (Advanced Paediatirc Life Support (APLS) 2004). If a choking episode is witnessed, interventions can commence immediately while the child is conscious. It is imperative that a clear history is obtained, as the choking algorithm must not be followed in children with signs of upper airway compromise due to illness, such as epiglottitis (Biarent *et al.* 2005).

Abdominal thrusts should not be used to treat choking infants because of the associated risk of causing intra-abdominal injury. Due to anatomical differences, infants who are in the horizontal position have their upper abdominal organs exposed to injury.

If the child is able to cough effectively (this includes being able to cry or the ability to answer questions, has a loud cough, is fully responsive or is able to take a breath before coughing) then he or she should be encouraged to do so while help is summoned. Continue to monitor the child closely.

If the child is conscious, but demonstrates absent or ineffective coughing (unable to talk, quiet or silent cough, unable to breathe, shows signs of cyanosis or shows a decreasing level of consciousness), back blows and chest thrusts in infants should be administered. In older children, back blows and abdominal thrusts should be performed until the object is removed.

Up to five back blows should be attempted in both infants and children, ideally the head should be lower than the chest in order to facilitate removal of the object. If this is not successful then the rescuer should attempt chest or abdominal thrusts.

For infants, perform up to five chest thrusts, again the head should be lower than the chest. The landmarks for chest thrusts are the same as for cardiac chest compressions; however, chest thrusts must be slower and more vigorous than chest compressions.

In the child up to five abdominal thrusts should also be performed. Standing behind the child, the rescuer places a fist in the child's epigastrium and the other hand pulls inwards and upwards sharply. The objective of all these manoeuvres is to increase intrathoracic pressure in order to expel the object. After each series of interventions, the child/infant should be reassessed in order to ascertain whether the foreign body is visible or their level of consciousness has decreased.

If the child or infant becomes unconscious, assess the airway to identify whether the object is visible and can be removed under direct vision. If this is not possible, the BLS algorithm should be followed commencing with five rescue breaths. Help should be summoned and the sequence repeated until the object is removed or expert help arrives (Resuscitation Council UK 2005).

Paediatric ALS infants and children (see Figure 8.8)

The majority of cardiac arrests in children are caused by respiratory or circulatory failure (Herlitz *et al.* 2005) although ventricular fibrillation (VF) may be the cause in 7–15% of infants and children (ILCOR 2005).

The priority in ALS is to ensure that adequate BLS is instituted and ongoing throughout the resuscitation attempt. Once effective BLS is ongoing with effective ventilation and high flow oxygen, a cardiac monitor should be attached so the cardiac rhythm can be assessed. No more than 10 seconds should be taken to assess the rhythm. The most common cardiac arrest rhythm is a non-shockable rhythm, either asystole or pulseless electrical activity (PEA) (see Chapter 11).

Asystole and PEA – non-shockable

The treatment of asystole and PEA is effective ventilation, using high concentration oxygen and a 2-minute cycle of cardiopulmonary resuscitation (CPR). Unless the rhythm changes to one which may support an output, performing a 10-second pulse check every 2 minutes should be avoided. Each time there is a pause in chest compressions, coronary perfusion pressure falls dramatically. Adrenaline (10 μg/kg) should be given at 3- to 5-minute intervals in order to

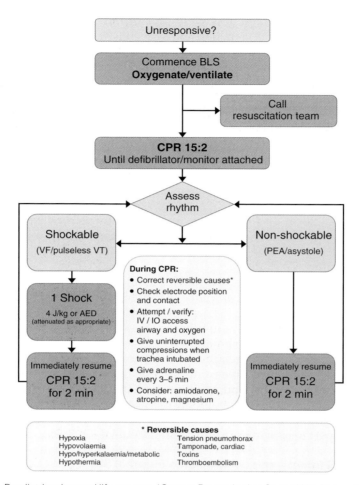

Figure 8.8 Paediatric advanced life support. (*Source*: Resuscitation Council UK, Resuscitation Guidelines 2005. Reproduced with kind permission of the Resuscitation Council UK.)

increase coronary perfusion pressure and enhance myocardial contractility. As soon as the child is intubated then asynchronous continuous compressions should be given at a rate of 100 per minute with ten ventilations/min. Any reversible causes should be identified and treated (four H's and four T's; see Chapter 13).

VF/pulseless VT – shockable
- The treatment of a shockable rhythm focuses on early defibrillation and effective BLS. A single shock of 4 J/kg should be delivered followed immediately by 2 minutes of CPR. After 2 minutes of CPR, analyse the rhythm using manual paddles or gel pads.
- A second shock at 4 J/kg should be delivered if VF/pulseless VT persists, CPR is immediately resumed for another 2 minutes

- Analyse cardiac rhythm; if there is no change, give a further 10 μg/kg of adrenaline immediately before the next shock at 4 J/kg is delivered.
- Immediately after repeat of 2 minutes of CPR, establish whether there is a shockable rhythm present.
- If a shockable rhythm continues, give 5 mg/kg of amiodarone followed immediately by a fourth shock.
- Continue with another 2 minutes of CPR before reviewing the cardiac rhythm.
- If a shockable rhythm remains, give adrenaline at 10 μg/kg immediately prior to the fifth shock. Monitor checks and defibrillation after 2 minutes of CPR are continued with adrenaline being administered at 3- to 5-minute intervals.

Defibrillation

Biphasic defibrillation

Biphasic defibrillators are increasingly being introduced into clinical practice. Biphasic shocks have been found to be at least as effective and produce less post-shock myocardial dysfunction than monophasic shocks (Faddy *et al.* 2003). As yet, there is little evidence to show the optimal energy to be used in biphasic defibrillation in children. The current recommendation is that 4 J/kg should be delivered to children in a shockable rhythm, whether a monophasic or biphasic defibrillator is used (Biarent *et al.* 2005).

Paddle size

In manual defibrillation, the largest paddles available should be used without touching them. In infants, the suggested optimum paddle size is 4.5 cm, and in children over 1 year old, the diameter suggested is 8–12 cm. The paddles should be firmly applied to the child's chest: one placed below the right clavicle and other in the left axilla. Hands free defibrillators are increasingly being used and appropriate-sized stick on pads are available.

Automated external defibrillators

Automated external defibrillators (AEDs) have been used to successfully defibrillate children under the age of eight years (Konig *et al.* 2005); as more evidence emerges, it has been found that AEDs are sensitive and accurate in identifying arrhythmias in children. It has been found that there is a very low risk of an inappropriate shock being advised. Attenuated AEDs are now available which are appropriate in the use of children between one and eight years old (energy levels of 50–75 J). The Resuscitation Council UK (2005) recommends that if no appropriate defibrillator is available then an AED delivering adult energy shocks may be used in children over one year.

Intraosseous access

Intravenous access can be extremely difficult to obtain in a child with poor or no cardiac output. The Resuscitation Council UK (2005) recommends that intraosseous (IO) access should be the first line of vascular access in the child who present in cardiac arrest with no vascular access.

Understanding the physiology of the IO route allows us to understand why it is such a good substitute for intravenous access in an emergency situation. The IO space is connected to the central circulation through a system of non-collapsible bony sinusoids and vessels. Drugs or fluids infused via the IO route enter a network of venous sinusoids within the medullary cavity; these drain into the central venous channels via nutrient or emissary veins (Blumberg *et al.* 2008, Evans *et al.* 1995). There is evidence to prove that the administration of drugs via the IO route will reach the central circulation in the same time when compared with the administration of intravenous drugs (VonHoff *et al.* 2008).

- Any drug or fluid can be infused via the IO route (with the exception of bretylium).
- The most common site for IO cannulation is the proximal tibia, the distal afemur; iliac crest and calcaneum have also been successfully used (McCarthy & Buss 1988).
- On insertion of the IO needle, a small amount of bone marrow (usually 1–2 mL) can be aspirated and sent for measurement of urea and electrolytes and glucose as well as cross matching.
- The IO route has been found to be a safe and fast technique to gain vascular access in emergency situations with <1% of complications being reported in patients (American Heart Association 2000).

Calculating drug doses and equipment sizes in paediatric resuscitation

Drug doses for children are based on their weight in order that therapeutic ranges are achieved and the child does not receive an over or under dose of drugs. In an emergency, it is difficult to ascertain an accurate weight, so formulae have been devised in order to help healthcare professionals work out a child's weight.

The formula (age + 4) × 2 can be used accurately between the age of one year and puberty; for example, a child who is two years old:

$$(2+4) \times 2 = 12\,\text{kg}$$

The advantage of this calculation is that it is simple to remember and calculate and does not require direct measurement of the child (Tinning & Acworth 2007).

A dose of 10 µg/kg of adrenaline should be administered every 3–5 minutes. This equates to 0.1 mL/kg of 1:10 000 adrenaline; thus, a child who weighs 20 kg should receive 2 mL of 110 000 adrenaline intravenously or via the IO route every 3–5 minutes.

Further formulae have been developed for calculating the correct equipment to use in children across a range of ages.

Internal diameter size of endotracheal tube in mm

$$(age/4) + 4$$

Length of oral endotracheal tube in cm

$$(age/2) + 12$$

Length of nasal endotracheal tube in cm

$$(age/2) + 15$$

(APLS 2004).

Family presence

There has been much debate in the literature in recent years over the advantages and disadvantages of family presence during the resuscitation attempts of their child. Bauchner *et al.* (1991) found that the majority of parents would like to be present during a resuscitation attempt of their child. Advantages of family presence include the fact that parents witnessing their child's resuscitation can see that everything possible has been attempted (Hanson & Strawser 1992). It also gives the family an opportunity to say goodbye to their child if the resuscitation was not successful and helps them to gain a realistic view of the resuscitation and the child's death (Meyers *et al.* 2000). There is evidence to suggest that families who were present at their child's death were able to begin the process of grieving and showed less anxiety and depression several months later when compared with families who were bereaved and had not been able to be present at their child's death (Robinson *et al.* 1998). Healthcare professionals have expressed concerns that parental presence during resuscitation attempts could be disruptive and not allow the team to concentrate on the resuscitation attempt; others have expressed concerns that parents would physically prevent the team from resuscitating the patient (Beckman *et al.* 2002). However, Meyers *et al.* (2000) suggested that parental presence may help healthcare professionals maintain professional behaviours as well as remembering that the child was part of a family.

Guidelines for staff need to be developed in areas where parental presence may occur during resuscitation attempts. Best practice suggests that a dedicated member of the resuscitation team should be present with the parents to explain the process and provide support during and after the resuscitation efforts (Biarent *et al.* 2005). A joint position statement on the presence of family members during cardiopulmonary resuscitation was published by the European Federation of Critical Care Nursing Associations together with the European Society of Paediatric and Neonatal Intensive Care and the European Society of Cardiology Council on Cardiovascular Nursing and Allied Professions (Fulbrook *et al.* 2007) (see Chapter 2).

Case study

A two-year-old child has been admitted to the paediatric intensive care unit following a respiratory arrest. The child has been successfully resuscitated and is admitted to the unit intubated and ventilated.

What size of ETT would you expect the child to require?

(answer: age/4 + 4 = 4.5 mm)

You are alerted to the alarms on the monitoring equipment, on assessing the child, there is no cardiac output. When you look at the cardiac monitor, which cardiac arrest rhythm are you most likely to see?

(answer: asystole)

What are the appropriate ratios of cardiac compressions to ventilations in this age child?

(answer: continuous asynchronous compressions at a rate of 100 per minute as the child is intubated and ventilated)

What is the dose of adrenaline required every 3–5 minutes during the resuscitation?

(answer: 10 μg/kg of 1:10 000 adrenaline = 2(age + 4) = 12 kg; so correct dose = 1.2 mL of 1:10 000 adrenaline IV)

How would you assess if the ETT was positioned in the correct place?

(answer: observe for symmetrical chest wall movement and auscultate the chest in the right and left mid-axilla).

What should be the next action if no breath sounds were heard in the right or left axilla?

(answer: remove the ETT and continue to ventilate the child using a bag-valve mask and ensure the chest wall was moving with each breath)

REVIEW OF LEARNING
Summary of basic life support.

	Infant	Child
Airway position	Neutral	Sniffing
Initial rescue breaths	5	5
Position of pulse check	Brachial/femoral	Carotid
Chest compression landmarks	One finger breadth above Xiphisternum	One finger breadth above Xiphisternum
Ratio of compression to ventilations	15:2	15:2
Compression rate	100 per min	100 per min

Review of learning ALS
The foundation of effective ALS is effective BLS. Assessment of the cardiac arrest rhythm is key as to the use of the appropriate cardiac arrest algorithm. The majority of children will present in a non-shockable rhythm, and the focus of this algorithm is good quality CPR (which should be continuous and asynchronous once the child is intubated) with adrenaline delivered every 3–5 minutes. It is essential that an estimation of a child's weight is made early on in the resuscitation so appropriate doses of drugs and energy are delivered.

CONCLUSION

While the outcome of paediatric cardiac arrest is poor, early assessment and intervention to prevent the child from deteriorating and arresting is key. However, if the child does present in cardiac arrest, the best available sequence of interventions for a positive outcome is produced in the current evidence-based paediatric ALS guidelines (Resuscitation Council UK 2005).

REFERENCES

Advanced Paediatric Life Support Group (APLS) (2004) *Advanced Paediatric Life Support: The Practical Approach*, 4th edn. BMJ Publishing Group, London.

American Heart Association (2000) Pediatric advanced life support. *Resuscitation* **46** (1–3), 343–99

Bauchner, H., Waring, C. & Vinci, R. (1991) Parental presence during procedures in an emergency room: results from 50 observations. *Pediatrics* **87**, 544–8.

Beckman, A.W., Sloan, B.K. & Moore, G.P. (2002) Should parents be present during emergency department procedures on children, and who should make that decision? A survey of emergency physician and nurse attitudes. *Academic Emergency Medicine* **9**, 154–8.

Berg, R.A., Hilwig, R.W., Kern, K.B. & Ewy, G.A. (2000) Bystander chest compressions and assisted ventilation independently improve outcome form piglet asphyxia pulseless cardiac arrest. *Circulation* **101**, 1743–8.

Biarent, D., Bingham, R., Richmond, S. *et al.* (2005) European Resuscitation Council guidelines for resuscitation 2005. Section 6. *Paediatric Life Support* **6751**, S97–133.

Blumberg, S., Gorn, M., & Crain, F. (2008) Intraosseous infusion: a review of methods and novel devices. *Paediatric Emergency Care* **24** (1), 50–56.

Byrne, E. & Phillips, B. (2003) The physiology behind resuscitation guidelines. *Current Paediatrics* **13** (1), 1–5.

Clements, F. & McGowan, J. (2000) Finger position for chest compressions in cardiac arrest in infants. *Resuscitation* **44**, 43–6.

Donoghue, A.J., Nadkarni, V., & Berg, R.A. (2005) Out of hospital pediatric cardiac arrest: an epidemiological review and assessment of current knowledge. *Annals of Emergency Medicine* **46** (6), 512–22.

Engdahl, J., Axelsson, A., Bang, A., Karlson, B.W. & Hertlitz J. (2003) The epidemiology of cardiac arrest in children and young adults. *Resuscitation* **58**, 131–8.

European Resuscitation Council (2005) European Resuscitation Council guidelines for resuscitation 2005. *Resuscitation* **67** (suppl 1), S1–190.

Evans, R.J., Jewkes, F., Owen, G., McCabe, M. & Palmer, D. (1995) Intraosseous infusion, a technique available for intravascular administration of drugs and fluids in the child with burns. *Burns* **21** (7), 552–3.

Faddy, S.C., Powell, J. & Craig, J.C. (2003) Biphasic and monophasic shocks for transthoracic defibrillation: a meta analysis of randomised controlled trials. *Resuscitation* **58**, 9–16.

Fulbrook, P., Latour, J., Albarran, J. *et al.*, for The Presence of Family Members During Cardiopulmonary Resuscitation Working Group (2007) The presence of family members during cardiopulmonary resuscitation: European Federation of Critical Care Nursing Associations, European Society of Paediatric and Neonatal Intensive Care and European Society of Cardiology Council on Cardiovascular Nursing and Allied Professions Joint Position Statement. *The World of Critical Care Nursing* **5** (4), 86–8.

Hanson, C. & Strawser, D. (1992) Family presence during cardiopulmonary resuscitation: Foote Hospital emergency department's nine year perspective. *Journal of Emergency Nursing* **18**, 104–6.

Herlitz, J., Engdahl, J., Svensson, L., Young, M., Angquist, K.A. & Holmberg, S. (2005) Characteristics and outcome among children suffering form out of hospital cardiac arrest in Sweden. *Resuscitation* **64**, 37–40.

International Liaison Committee on Resuscitation (ILCOR) (2005) Paediatric basic and advanced life support. *Resuscitation* **67**, 271–91.

Kinney, S.B. & Tibballs, J. (1999) An analysis of the efficacy of bag-valve-mask ventilation and chest compression. *Resuscitation* **30** (2), 141–50.

Konig, B., Benger, J. & Goldsworthy, L. (2005) Automatic external defibrillation in a 6 year old. *Archives of Diseases in Children* **90**, 310–11.

McCarthy, G. & Buss, P. (1988) The calcaneum as a site for IO infusion. *Journal of Accident and Emergency Medicine* **15** (6), 421–9.

Meyers, T.A., Eichhorn, D.J. & Guzzetta, C.E. (2000) Family presence during invasive procedures and resuscitation. *American Journal of Nursing* **100**, 32–42.

Resuscitation Council UK (RC UK) (2005) *Resuscitation Guidelines 2005*. RC UK, London.

Robinson, S.M., Mackenzie-Ross, S., Campbell Hewson, G.L., Egleston, C.V. & Prevost, A.T. (1998) Psychological effect of witnessed resuscitation on bereaved relatives. *Lancet* **352**, 614–17.

Tinning, K. & Acworth, J. (2007) Make your best guess: an updated method for paediatric weight estimate in emergencies. *Emergency Medicine Australasia* **19**, 528–34.

VonHoff, D., Kuhn, J., Burris, H. & Miller, L. (2008) Does intraosseous equal intravenous? A pharmacokinetic study. *The American Journal of Emergency Medicine* **26**, 31–8.

Section 6

Further Considerations of Resuscitation

Una McKay

9 | Management of the Airway and Breathing

INTRODUCTION
Good airway management is an essential part of basic life support (BLS) and advanced life support (ALS). In a patient who is breathing spontaneously, supplemental oxygen may prevent a cardiac or respiratory arrest. Any person in respiratory distress or cardiovascular crisis should also receive supplemental oxygen. During cardiac arrest, it is impossible to restart the heart without adequate oxygenation. Recognising airway and breathing problems promptly and responding with appropriate interventions will ensure hypoxic damage to vital organs is minimised.

AIMS
This chapter considers the management of airway and breathing in the compromised patient.

LEARNING OUTCOMES
At the end of the chapter, the reader will be able to:

❏ discuss *potential causes* of airway obstruction;
❏ recognise airway problems using a *systematic assessment*;
❏ respond to airway and breathing problems with *appropriate interventions*;
❏ appreciate *advanced airway and breathing issues*.

REVIEW OF THE NORMAL AIRWAY
The airway is divided into the upper airway and the lower airway. The upper airway comprises the nose, mouth and pharynx. The lower airway comprises the larynx, trachea and lungs. During normal breathing, oxygenated air enters the lungs through an open airway and oxygenates the blood. This is transported to the tissues providing the circulation is adequate. A lack of oxygen causes tissue hypoxia. Some organs are more sensitive to hypoxia. For example, if deprived of oxygen even for a short period of time, the brain is adversely affected. The patient may become agitated or confused and eventually his or her level of consciousness will deteriorate, leading to potentially irreversible or fatal brain damage.

Carbon dioxide is exhaled in normal breathing. An airway obstruction or breathing difficulty may result in the build-up of carbon dioxide in the blood (hypercarbia), and the patient may appear drowsy or lethargic.

Table 9.1 Common causes of airway obstruction.

Level of obstruction		Potential causes
Upper airway	Mouth, nose, pharynx (often referred to nasopharynx, oropharynx and hypopharynx)	Most common – loss of pharyngeal muscle tone; vomit, blood, foreign body; epiglottis swelling; soft tissue oedema
Lower airway	Larynx	Oedema, laryngospasm (spasm of vocal cords); foreign body, trauma
	Trachea	Secretions or foreign body; swelling
	Lungs (the trachea branches into the right and left bronchi; lower passageways are called bronchioles)	Bronchospasm; pulmonary oedema; aspiration

AIRWAY OBSTRUCTION

Airway obstruction frequently occurs in the critically ill or injured patient (Cook & Hommers 2006). The obstruction may be either the result of, or may cause, loss of consciousness. The patient may have partial or complete obstruction and it may occur anywhere from the nose and mouth down to the bronchi (see Table 9.1). The tongue is the most common cause of airway obstruction in the unresponsive casualty (Baskett *et al.* 1996).

Recognising an airway problem

The best way to recognise a partial or complete airway obstruction is by looking, listening and feeling (Baskett *et al.* 1996).

Look

- The patient who is able to verbalise clearly has an airway that is patent and not compromised at this point.
- An agitated and/or confused patient may be hypoxic.
- A lethargic patient may be hypercarbic.
- A cyanotic and pale patient is likely to be hypoxic. The skin may also be clammy or sweaty. Note that cyanosis is often a late sign and absence of cyanosis does not mean that the patient is adequately oxygenated.
- A patient showing signs of muscular retractions, who is making use of his or her accessory muscles or has shallow, laboured breathing has some degree of airway compromise.

Listen

- A patient whose respiration is quiet and effortless is breathing normally.
- Noisy breathing indicates partial airway obstruction (see Table 9.2).
- If there are no breath sounds, this indicates the absence of air entry that may be due to complete airway obstruction.

Table 9.2 Obstructive airway sounds.

Characteristic sounds	What they mean
Crowing	Laryngeal spasm or obstruction
Wheeze	An expiratory noise suggestive of lower airway obstruction
Stridor	An inspiratory noise suggestive of upper airway obstruction
Gurgling	Suggestive of liquid or semisolid foreign material in the main airways
Snoring	Indicates the pharynx is partially occluded by the tongue or palate

Feel
- A patient whose chest is moving equally and quietly, exhaling warm air, is breathing normally.
- If air cannot be felt but chest and abdominal movements are obvious, this is indicative of complete airway obstruction.

Basic airway opening techniques

Basic airway opening manoeuvres are simple techniques that can be performed anywhere and without the use of equipment. In most situations, the commonly used techniques of head tilt/chin lift and/or jaw thrust may be all that is required to relieve airway obstruction caused by the relaxation of soft tissues. These very basic manoeuvres are described as part of BLS in Chapter 6.

- It is imperative that once a manoeuvre has been performed, it must not be assumed that it has been successful in opening the airway.
- Assessment should continue, using the look, listen and feel approach.
- If it is not possible to achieve a clear airway using either of these manoeuvres, it may be necessary to consider the use of suction or a simple airway adjunct.
- If there is evidence of trauma or any reason to suspect cervical spine injury, the jaw thrust is the airway opening technique of choice (International Liaison Committee on Resuscitation (ILCOR) 2005).

Oropharyngeal suctioning

The patient may have liquid (gastric contents, saliva, blood) present in the upper airway. This has the potential to cause airway obstruction or aspiration and therefore needs to be removed from the upper airway as quickly as possible.

There are a variety of suction devices available to assist in clearing the upper airway. The commonest device is a wide-bore rigid sucker (Yankauer), which is attached to a suction apparatus. Important points to remember are:

- the rescuer should always wear gloves when suctioning the patient;
- to perform oropharyngeal suctioning, the suction device should be carefully inserted into the patient's mouth. The tip of the suction device should be visible at all times to avoid stimulating a gag reflex.

Figure 9.1 illustrates a Yankauer sucker and suction unit.

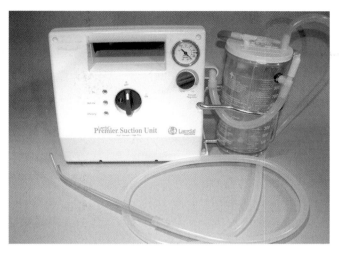

Figure 9.1 Battery-operated suction device with Yankaeur suction catheter attached.

AIRWAY ADJUNCTS

Airway adjuncts help improve and maintain an open and patent airway. Commonly used adjuncts include pharyngeal airways, such as the oropharyngeal airway and nasopharyngeal airway. Both of these adjuncts can be used in the patient who is unconscious and is stopped breathing. In this situation, the adjuncts help maintain airway patency during the use of ventilatory devices such as the pocket mask or bag-valve-mask system (ILCOR 2005). The unconscious patient who is stopped breathing may also benefit from the insertion of a supraglottic airway device such as a laryngeal mask airway (LMA) or combitube, both of which offer a more secure airway when personnel skilled in endotracheal intubation are not immediately available (Stone *et al*. 1998).

Pharyngeal airways

The oropharyngeal and nasopharyngeal airways are devices that help to prevent backward displacement of the tongue in an unconscious patient. It is important to note that a degree of head tilt, chin lift or jaw thrust may still be necessary when using an airway adjunct (ILCOR 2005). The patient who has an oropharyngeal or nasopharyngeal airway in situ but is breathing spontaneously will require supplemental oxygen via a delivery system (as described in Chapter 3). Failure to administer oxygen to seriously ill patients will compromise their chances of survival.

Oropharyngeal airway

For details on equipment design and indications for use, refer to Chapter 4.

Sizing
- Estimate the correct size by holding the airway vertically between the angle of the jaw and the incisors (as shown in Figure 9.2).

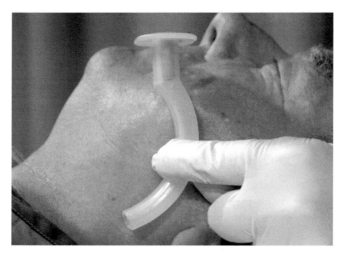

Figure 9.2 Correct sizing of an oropharyngeal airway.

- An incorrectly sized airway, one that is too long or too short, may further obstruct the patient's airway or be ineffective.

Insertion technique (see Figures 9.3(a)–9.3(c))
- Open the patient's mouth and ensure it is clear of any debris or foreign material.
- Insert the airway into the mouth in what initially appears to be the 'upside down' position until it is approximately halfway inserted.
- Rotate the airway 180° and continue to push it into place in the oral cavity. The reinforced section should sit firmly between the patient's teeth with the flange to the outside of the lips. If the patient does not have teeth, the reinforced section should rest between the gums.
- Assess the patient for airway and breathing, using the look, listen and feel sequence.

Nasopharyngeal airway
For details on equipment design and indications for use, refer to Chapter 4.

Sizing
- Sizes for this airway indicate the internal diameter in millimetres. As diameter size increases, so does the length.
- Most adults require a size 6 or 7 but sizes 8 and 9 are also available.
- A tube that is too long may enter the oesophagus or may cause laryngospasm and vomiting.

Insertion technique (see Figures 9.4(a)–9.4(b))
- Check patency of the patient's nostrils. Generally, the right nostril is preferred.

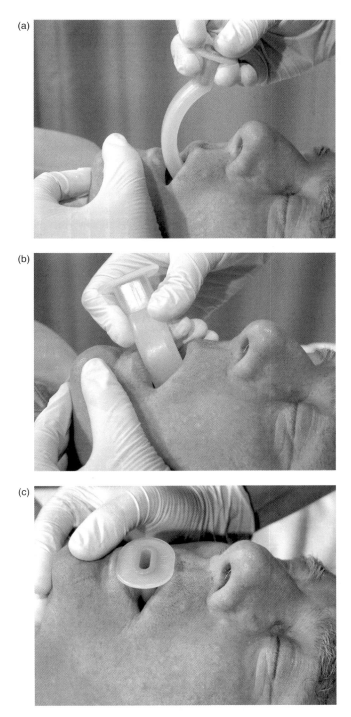

Figure 9.3 Insertion of an oropharyngeal airway.

(a)

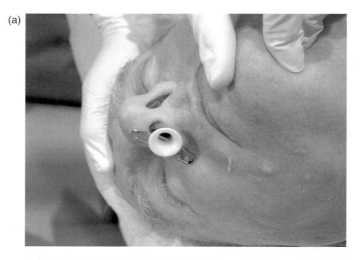

(b)

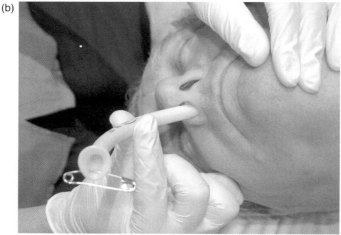

Figure 9.4 Insertion of a nasopharyngeal airway.

- Ensure that the airway is well lubricated with a water-soluble jelly. Some nasopharyngeal airways also require the insertion of a safety pin at the trumpet end to give extra protection against the airway slipping beyond the nostril.
- Insert the angular end into the patient's nostril and slide the airway along the floor of the nose by using a small twisting motion (in a patient who is supine, this is in a downward vertical direction).
- If there is any obstruction, try inserting the airway into the left nostril.
- Assess the patient for airway and breathing using the look, listen and feel sequence.
- Injury to the nasal mucosa may occur during insertion, leading to bleeding or problems when removing the airway. Always be prepared with suction to remove secretions or blood.

Supraglottic airway devices

Supraglottic airway devices are now used widely during routine surgery (Richez *et al.* 2008) and have revolutionised airway management during general anaesthesia (Cook & Hommers 2006). Their ease of use make them potentially useful during resuscitation. At present, the International Liason Committee on Resuscitation (ILCOR 2005) only recommend the LMA and combitube in its guidelines. However, a new supraglottic airway device, the 'I-Gel', is presently receiving much attention as it has some distinct features (such as increased ease of insertion and not requiring inflation with any air), which set it apart from many of its competitors (Gabbott & Beringer 2007). Whilst the use of the I-Gel during resuscitation does look extremely promising, it is important to stress that devices need to have a sound evidence base prior to recommending widespread use (Soar 2007).

Laryngeal mask airway

For details on equipment design and indications for use, refer to Chapter 4. The LMA may be inserted almost immediately in the patient who has stopped breathing and become deeply unconscious.

There is some evidence to suggest that when a bag-valve device is used to ventilate the patient prior to insertion of the LMA, gastric regurgitation and aspiration are more likely to occur than if the LMA has been inserted immediately, without prior ventilation, as a first-line airway adjunct (Stone *et al.* 1998).

Once a ventilatory device such as a bag-valve is attached to the LMA, it is important that high inflation pressures are not generated during ventilation as this increases the risk of gastric inflation and therefore potential regurgitation and aspiration.

Sizing

- The LMA is available in sizes suitable for neonates through to large adults.
- A size 4 or 5 is suitable for all but very small adults, who may be more suited to a size 3.

Insertion technique (see Figures 9.5(a)–9.5(c))

- Check the cuff patency by inserting the appropriate amount of air (as shown in Table 9.3). Deflate the cuff and ensure the outer face of the cuff is lubricated.
- Position the patient supine with the head and neck aligned. Slightly flex the neck and extend the head unless there is suspicion of cervical spine injury.
- Hold the tube like a pen and introduce the cuff into the patient's mouth. Using the index finger to provide support at the tip of the cuff, advance it along

Table 9.3 LMA cuff inflation volumes.

LMA size	Patient size	Cuff inflation
3	Small adult	Up to 20 mL
4	Medium adult	Up to 30 mL
5	Large adult	Up to 40 mL

(a)

(b)

(c)

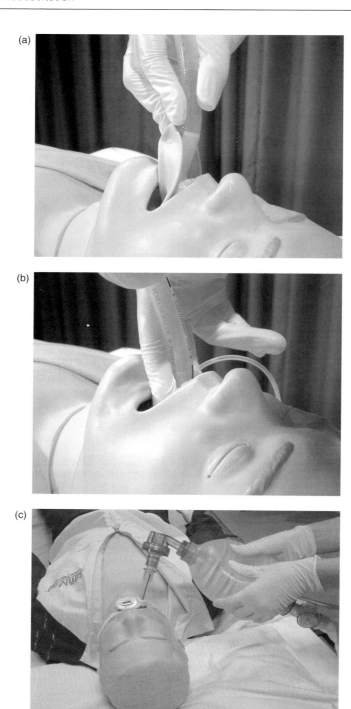

Figure 9.5 Insertion of an LMA.

the roof of the patient's mouth into the airway until it reaches the back of the throat.

- Take hold of the external part of the tube and, keeping it in the midline, advance it further until resistance is felt and it locates in the back of the pharynx.
- Inflate the cuff with the appropriate amount of air. The tube should lift 1–2 cm out of the mouth as the cuff finds its correct position on inflation.
- Connect the tube to a bag-valve device with supplemental oxygen and confirm adequate ventilation by noting bilateral chest movement. Use a stethoscope to listen for air entry during ventilation.
- If placement of the LMA does not allow adequate ventilation within 30 seconds of commencement, it should be removed and the patient ventilated and oxygenated prior to further attempts.
- Insert a bite block, such as a roll of gauze or oropharyngeal airway, alongside the tube and tie the tube securely.

Combitube

At the time of writing, the combitube is not widely used in the UK, in contrast to North America and many parts of Europe (ILCOR 2005). However, it is worth a brief mention as it offers similar appeal to the LMA in terms of training and skill requirements.

The combitube is a rigid double-lumen tube that is inserted blindly into the patient's mouth and advanced towards the larynx. In the majority of cases the tube enters the patient's oesophagus but the design of the tube caters for the occasion when it may directly enter the trachea. The combitube has a series of perforations and inflatable cuffs and due to the double lumen, the healthcare professional trained in its use would assess which port to ventilate by, depending on whether the device had lodged itself in the oesophagus or trachea. The combitube and equipment necessary for its insertion are as shown in Figure 9.6.

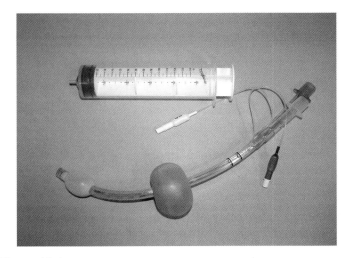

Figure 9.6 The combitube.

VENTILATION

The patient who is not breathing or breathing inadequately will require assisted ventilation (Wenzel *et al.* 2001). This can be achieved by:

- mouth-to-mouth (nose) ventilation;
- mouth-to-mask ventilation;
- bag-valve device (attached to facemask, laryngeal mask airway, combitube, endotracheal tube);
- automatic, mechanical ventilators.

Mouth-to-mouth (nose) ventilation

Simple barrier devices such as faceshields are available to prevent direct mouth-to-mouth (nose) contact (Wenzel *et al.* 2001). These are usually plastic or silicone sheet-type devices that often have a one-way valve system. Some of them have a small tube that should be inserted into the patient's mouth whilst ensuring that it is not obstructed by the tongue. Mouth-to-faceshield breathing is continued in the same manner as mouth-to-mouth breathing (see Chapter 6).

Mouth-to-mask ventilation

The pocket mask is an excellent device that allows effective ventilation of a patient by less experienced personnel (Baskett *et al.* 1996). The mask provides protection to the rescuer through a one-way valve system. The pocket resuscitation mask is an anatomically shaped facemask with a cushioned under-edge. Most are marked to guide positioning of the mask on the patient's face. Some masks have an oxygen inlet, which allows supplemental oxygen to be given in addition to the rescuer's breaths. If no oxygen inlet is present, supplemental oxygen may still be administered by placing the oxygen tubing directly under the mask. There must be a good seal between the mask and the patient's face.

Technique

Ideally, the patient should be in a supine position.

- Remove the mask from its container and form it into the correct shape by pushing the dome part forward (see Figures 9.7(a)–9.7(b)).
- Attach the one-way valve to the mouthpiece.
- Wear the gloves that are provided in the pocket mask container.
- Standing beside the patient or behind the patient's head, apply the mask to the patient's face. Use the bridge of the nose as a guide for correct placement.
- Apply firm pressure onto the cushioned part of the mask using your fingers and/or thumbs in a position that is comfortable and ensures a good seal between the mask and the patient's face.
- Perform head tilt/chin lift to open the airway.
- Blow gently through the one-way valve and look for chest movement. The chest should rise as with normal breathing. It is not necessary for the rescuer to deliver large breaths to effectively ventilate the patient's lungs.

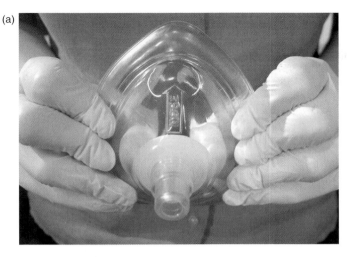

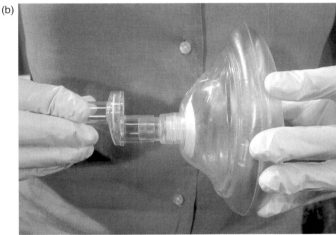

Figure 9.7 Assembly of pocket mask.

- Allow the patient to exhale between each ventilation. Watch for the chest to fall before giving the next breath.
- Be aware that it may be difficult to get an adequate seal on the first attempt. In this situation, reposition fingers and thumbs, adjust the mask and be sure the airway is opened correctly.
- An oral airway may be used to assist in maintaining the airway when using the pocket mask. However, attempted ventilation should not be delayed if one is not immediately available.
- Once oxygen is available, it should be attached to the oxygen inlet at a flow rate of 10 L/min. It is still necessary for the rescuer to blow into the mask to provide ventilation (see Figure 9.8).

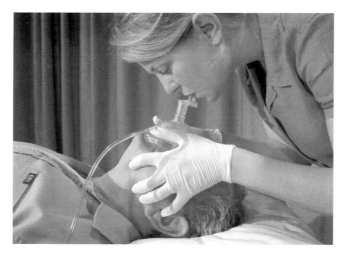

Figure 9.8 Mouth-to-mask ventilation with additional oxygen attached.

Bag-valve device

Different sized facemasks
- The facial anatomy of casualties always varies and so it is important to have a selection of suitable facemask sizes. The facemask should attach to the bag-valve system and a good seal need to be achieved for effective ventilation.
- The facemasks should be made of clear material so that the operator may observe any blood or vomit coming from the patient's airway.

Technique
A two-person technique is recommended when using the bag-valve device with a facemask (Resuscitation Council UK 2006). One rescuer should hold the mask securely in place whilst maintaining a head tilt/chin lift position. The second rescuer should squeeze the bag gently to inflate the casualty's lungs (see Figure 9.9).

The recommended tidal volumes for ventilations given with a bag-valve device with supplemental oxygen are 6–7 mL/kg (Resuscitation Council UK 2006). This tidal volume should provide normal chest movement in the casualty. Table 9.4 offers a guide for delivering supplementary oxygen.

Automatic mechanical ventilators
Automatic mechanical ventilators may be a useful adjunct during cardiopulmonary resuscitation, particularly in the pre-hospital setting where rescue times will be longer.

The ventilator is a small device that is often powered by the same oxygen cylinder which supplies the patient with oxygen. It works by providing a constant flow of gas to the patient during inspiration and has in-built pressure limitation controls. Considerable training is required and its use would therefore not be appropriate for an occasional user (Resuscitation Council UK 2006).

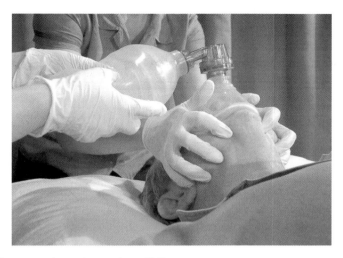

Figure 9.9   Two-person bag-valve-mask ventilation.

ADVANCED AIRWAY CONTROL AND VENTILATION: TRACHEAL INTUBATION

Intubation of the trachea with a cuffed tube is still considered to be the best possible means of maintaining a clear and secure airway in the cardiac arrest casualty (ILCOR 2005). However, whether or not this will result in an improved chance of survival for the adult casualty has not yet been proven through a prospective randomised trial. Tracheal intubation should be used only when trained personnel are available to carry out the procedure with a high level of skill and confidence (Resuscitation Council UK 2006). The current ALS algorithm (see Chapter 7) emphasises the need for airway management and delivery of oxygen but it does not specify that intubation is absolutely necessary. In the absence of personnel skilled in intubation, there are acceptable alternatives, such as bag-valve-mask ventilation or the use of an LMA.

Table 9.4   Oxygen delivery guide.

Ventilatory device	Oxygen flow rate	Approximate oxygen concentration
Mouth-to-mouth (or nose)	Nil	16–17%
Mouth-to-mask	Nil	16–17%
Mouth-to-mask	10 L/min	40% or more
Bag-valve-mask (with no reservoir system attached)	Nil	21%
Bag-valve-mask (with reservoir system attached)	10–15 L/min	85%
Bag-valve-tube (LMA, ETT, combitube) with reservoir system attached	10–15 L/min	Up to 100%

Advantages of tracheal intubation
- Isolates the airway and prevents foreign material from entering the oropharynx.
- Provides a means of suctioning inhaled debris from the lower airway.
- Ventilation can generally be achieved without leaks, even if there is airway resistance.
- Prescribed tidal volumes can be delivered.
- It can be used as an alternative route to administer drugs if intravenous access is not achieved.

Disadvantages of tracheal intubation
- Intubation requires extensive training and regular practice to maintain the skill.
- Numerous complications can arise as a result of tracheal intubation being attempted by unskilled operators, such as ventilation being withheld for unacceptable periods whilst intubation is repeatedly 'attempted'. Failure to oxygenate and ventilate results in death.
- It is important that any healthcare professional who may assist with intubation is fully conversant with the equipment necessary for this procedure (see Chapter 4).

REVIEW OF LEARNING
- ❏ Recognising airway and breathing problems promptly and responding with appropriate interventions will ensure hypoxic damage to vital organs is minimised.
- ❏ Airway obstruction may be partial or complete. The tongue is the most common form of airway obstruction in a patient with a decreased level of consciousness.
- ❏ The best way to recognise any degree of airway obstruction is to assess the patient by looking, listening and feeling.
- ❏ Often the basic airway opening manoeuvres of head tilt, chin lift and jaw thrust may be all that is required to relieve airway obstruction caused by the tongue.
- ❏ Oropharyngeal and nasopharyngeal airways are simple adjuncts that help to prevent backward displacement of the tongue in an unconscious patient.
- ❏ The LMA is an extremely reliable device that can be used during a resuscitation attempt for a patient who has become unconscious and stopped breathing.
- ❏ Assisted ventilation can be achieved by several methods including mouth-to-mouth or nose, mouth-to-mask, bag-valve device attached to facemask, LMA or endotracheal tube or automatic mechanical ventilator.
- ❏ Where possible, oxygen should be administered with any ventilation attempts. Failure to do so may compromise chances of survival.
- ❏ The best way to ensure adequate ventilation in the patient is to assess by looking, listening and feeling.

Case study

Mrs Betty Booth is a 68-year-old lady who has been admitted to the ward for observation. She has taken an overdose of sedative drugs. Considering her diagnosis, this patient may be at risk for airway and breathing compromise.

Make a list of potential causes of airway and breathing difficulties in such a patient. In addition, discuss how you would recognise any deterioration in Mrs Booth's condition.

- Central nervous system depression following the overdose may result in loss of airway control;
- Hypoxia;
- Vomiting;
- Regurgitation of gastric contents;
- Loose dentures;
- Saliva.

The best way to recognise an airway or breathing problem is to:

- *look* for signs of a clear airway, level of responsiveness, skin colour and evidence of laboured breathing;
- *listen* to determine whether the patient's breathing is noisy, silent or effortless and quiet;
- *feel* for signs of exhaled air.

Following your assessment of Mrs Booth, you find that she is now difficult to arouse. She is pale and clammy with shallow breathing at a rate of approximately six breaths/min. You can hear gurgling coming from her airway.

How would you respond?
- Open the airway using head tilt and chin lift.
- Use suction to clear the mouth.
- Administer high-flow oxygen via a non-rebreather oxygen mask.
- Consider inserting an oropharyngeal or nasopharyngeal airway.
- Consider calling the medical emergency team.

Whilst you are managing the situation, you recognise that Mrs Booth has become completely unresponsive and has stopped breathing. A pulse check reveals bradycardia at 45 beats/min.

How will you respond to this further deterioration?
Call for appropriate help. If an LMA is immediately available and you are competent in its use then insert it without pre-oxygenation. If the LMA is not an option then begin to ventilate the patient using a mouth-to-mask or bag-valve-mask technique with supplemental oxygen attached. Aim to provide ventilations at a normal respiratory rate (approximately 12 breaths/min). Monitor the effectiveness of ventilations using the look, listen and feel approach. Consider further monitoring, i.e. pulse oximetry and electrocardiogram, to recognise any further deterioration in the circulatory system. Whilst the patient is in respiratory arrest, continue to check the pulse every minute.

CONCLUSION

This chapter considers the management of airway and breathing in the compromised casualty. The guidelines for delivery are designed to aid recall and support effective resuscitation and all healthcare professionals should be familiar with the most up-to-date guidelines, by regularly accessing the *Resuscitation* journal and Resuscitation Council UK and European Resuscitation Council websites (www.resus.org.uk and www.erc.edu).

REFERENCES

Baskett, P.J.F., Bossaert, L., Chamberlain, D. *et al.* (1996) Guidelines for the basic management of the airway and ventilation during resuscitation. A statement by the Airway and Ventilation Management Working Group of the European Resuscitation Council. *Resuscitation* **31**, 187–200.

Cook, T.M. & Hommers, C. (2006) New airways for Resuscitation? *Resuscitation* **69**, 371–87.

Gabbott, D.A. & Beringer, R. (2007) Letters to the editor. The I-Gel supraglottic airway: a potential role for resuscitation? *Resuscitation* **73**, 161–4.

International Liaison Committee on Resuscitation (2005) International consensus on cardiopulmonary resuscitation and emergency cardiovascular care science with treatment recommendations. Part 4: advanced life support. *Resuscitation* **67** (2–3), 213–47.

Resuscitation Council UK (2006) *Advanced Life Support Course Provider Manual*, 5th edn. Resuscitation Council UK, London.

Richez, B., Saltel, L., Banchereau, F., Torrielli, R. & Cross, A.M. (2008) A new single use supraglottic airway device with a noninflatable cuff and esophageal vent: an observational study of the I-Gel. *Anesthesia and Analgesia* **106** (4), 1137–9.

Soar, J. (2007) Letters to the editor: The I-Gel supraglottic airway and resuscitation – some initial thoughts. *Resuscitation* **74**, 197–9.

Stone, B.J., Chantler, P.J. & Baskett, P.J.F. (1998) The incidence of regurgitation during cardiopulmonary resuscitation: a comparison between the bag valve mask and laryngeal mask airway. *Resuscitation* **3**, 3–7.

Wenzel, V., Idris, A.H., Dorges, V. *et al.* (2001) The respiratory system during resuscitation: a review of the history, risk of infection during assisted ventilation, respiratory mechanics, and ventilation strategies for patients with an unprotected airway. *Resuscitation* **49**, 123–34.

Monitoring and Assessing Cardiac Rhythms

10

John W. Albarran

INTRODUCTION

Increasingly, healthcare staff are expected to manage the care of patients who may be at risk of developing life-threatening arrhythmias. To recognise and respond to life-threatening arrhythmias demands skill and knowledge as well as understanding of the effects that non-cardiac disorders have on the electrocardiograph (ECG).

Interpreting normal and abnormal cardiac rhythms requires detailed appreciation of the conducting system. In becoming familiar with the underlying concepts of electrocardiography and cardiac monitoring techniques, healthcare professionals can start to accurately differentiate rhythm disturbances that may suggest compromised cardiovascular function, myocardial irritability or instability which may precipitate a cardiac arrest.

AIMS

This chapter introduces the concepts associated with cardiac monitoring and discusses each of the main shockable, non-shockable and peri-arrest rhythms.

LEARNING OUTCOMES

By the end of this chapter, the reader will be able to:

❑ describe the *electrical conduction system of the heart*;
❑ discuss the *principles of cardiac monitoring*;
❑ explain the *main components of sinus rhythm*;
❑ describe the *physiological characteristics of shockable rhythms* and treatments;
❑ describe the *physiological characteristics of non-shockable rhythms and peri-arrest rhythms* and respective treatments.

ELECTRICAL CONDUCTION PATHWAYS OF THE HEART

Understanding the electrical activity of the heart is key to developing an appreciation of changes in the ECG.

Conducting system

• Electrical activity begins with pacemaker cells of the sinoatrial (SA) node. Here, cells are able to generate a spontaneous impulse without nervous innervation and normally determine the heart rate.

- Once the SA node depolarises, waves of electrical activity travel across the right and left atria, causing these chambers to contract.
- The impulses then reach the atrioventricular (AV) node, where there is a brief period of delayed conduction.
- Impulses are then propagated downwards in a coordinated fashion, initially along the AV bundle of His.
- The bundle consists of specialised conducting tissue that divides into the right and left bundle branches.
- The bundle of His and bundle branches are central to the propagation of impulses, which eventually terminate in fine branches or Purkinje fibres.
- The Purkinje fibres are embedded in ventricular myocardium and these will transmit impulses to the ventricular muscle mass, resulting in contraction. Ventricles comprise a large muscle mass and are able to generate spontaneous impulses but at a slower rate than pacemaker cells, namely at a rate of 20–40 beats/min (bpm) (Meek & Morris 2000a).

The spread of impulses from cell to cell and across the entire heart is known as 'depolarisation', whereas the stage of 'repolarisation' relates to myocardial recovery. In practice, the 'electrical' cycle of the heart can be fully assessed by a 12-lead ECG from the patient. Specifically, an ECG machine measures and records, on graph-like paper, voltage variations (of the atria and ventricles) plotted against time. These waves of electrical activity have three distinctive features.

Duration
The time element is measured along the horizontal axis and in fractions of a second:

- 1 small square equals 0.04 second or 1 mm in width;
- 1 large square equals 0.2 second or 5 mm in width;
- 300 large squares represent 1 minute.

Amplitude
A voltage component is measured along the vertical axis in millivolts:

- 1 small square equals 0.1 mV or 1 mm;
- 1 large square equals 0.5 mV or 5 mm.

Composition
This relates to specific arrangements in the waves in terms of shape and appearance.

PRINCIPLES OF CARDIAC MONITORING

The ECG displayed on the monitor screen must be clear and well defined to avoid misdiagnosis or inappropriate treatment. A cardiac trace can be obtained through three or five colour-coded ECG leads that are attached to electrodes placed on the anterior surface of a patient's chest. Signals emitted from the heart are sensed from the skin surface by the electrodes and are subsequently transmitted, by means of a cable, to the cardiac monitor, which in turn magnifies them into recognisable waves. The displayed image reflects one view and while

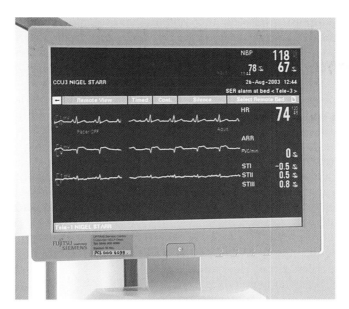

Figure 10.1 Monitor displays three leads and ST segment monitoring.

single-lead monitoring remains widely used, it has limited value in the diagnosis of other clinical conditions. However, modern monitors are multipurpose and permit a range of functions including continuous transmission of leads I, II and III (see Figure 10.1), as well as displaying non-invasive blood pressure and oxygen saturation readings. It is also possible to configure the technology to display 12-lead ECG and ST segment monitoring options.

Defibrillator paddles and gel pads can also be used to monitor a cardiac rhythm, particularly when the cardiac arrest is not witnessed. It is the quickest way to assess whether the casualty is in a shockable rhythm. Automated external defibrillators require application of large adhesive multipurpose electrodes to the casualty's chest, which allow for monitoring of cardiac rhythm and defibrillation.

Lead placement

For the purposes of monitoring, lead II should be selected as it provides the clearest view of the P wave and the QRS complex. A lead II trace is obtained by placing the red (positive) electrode on the right shoulder, the yellow (negative) electrode on the left shoulder and the black or green (neutral) electrode below the left border of the ribcage.

To ensure a high-quality ECG trace, consider the following principles:

- Maintain good skin contact (remove chest hair as it may interfere with adhesion of electrodes to skin).
- Keep skin surface dry (rub the sites selected for placement of electrodes with dry gauze).
- Apply even pressure only on adhesive area to ensure a good seal.
- Avoid placing electrodes where defibrillation gel pads might be positioned in the event of a cardiac arrest.

- Avoid interference from patient movement, electrical equipment and during cardiopulmonary resuscitation (CPR) by attaching the ECG electrodes over bone rather than muscle.
- Apply large adhesive multipurpose electrodes as recommended.
- Check ECG or replace electrodes if trace is poor or interrupted.
- Set alarms for upper and lower limits of heart rate in line with local practice.
- Record the patient's details, symptoms, date and time alongside the trace or ECG recording.

Problems encountered during cardiac monitoring
There are many factors that may affect the quality of the ECG trace appearing on the cardiac monitor so knowing how to minimise or prevent such problems is vital (Jevon 2003). Good practice involves always assessing the patient first before the equipment.

Straight/flat-line
- Assess for evidence of cable damage.
- Check that all equipment is connected correctly.
- Ensure the gain has been set appropriately.
- Make sure lead II has been selected.
- Check electrodes are in date and intact.
- Check other leads.

Quality of the ECG trace is inadequate
- Review connections and cable.
- Assess that electrodes have been correctly placed.
- Check that the electrodes have not become displaced.
- Electrodes are in date and intact.
- Replace electrodes.

Wandering baseline and artefacts
- Voluntary artefact – this can be caused by patient movement such as respiration. Consider moving electrodes.
- Involuntary artefact – this includes interference caused by shivering or nervousness. Keep patient warm and provide emotional support.
- Electrical interference – this is due to electrical equipment such as infusion pumps and syringe drivers. Ensure minimal contact with cardiac leads.
- Loose electrode – a wandering baseline pattern suggests signal interruption due to a loose electrode, poor contact or incorrectly placed electrode.
- Complexes are too small – these may be due to clinical factors such as a cardiac tamponade or pericardial effusion. Select a different lead, increase amplitude or substitute electrodes.
- False heart rate on display – occasionally the ECG complexes appear as very small on the cardiac monitor, giving the impression of a reduced heart rate. At other times the T wave may be counted for an R wave, thus doubling the heart rate. Reposition electrodes or select another lead to correct this problem (Jevon 2003).

COMPONENTS OF SINUS RHYTHM

Heart rate
Heart rate can be influenced by sympathetic and parasympathetic activity. Other factors that influence the heart rate include stimulants (nicotine, caffeine), drugs (beta-blockers) and conditions such as thyrotoxicosis and hypoxia. In health, the heart's resting rhythm is regular although the rate varies between 60 and 99 bpm (Meek & Morris 2002a).

Rhythm
Sinus rhythm is the term given to a rhythm that is regular and originates in the SA node, with a heart rate of 60–99 bpm. Sinus bradycardia is similar but the rate is below 60 whereas with sinus tachycardia, the rate is between 100 and 130 bpm.

Characteristic features of sinus rhythm
- The P wave is produced by atrial depolarisation. As the atria possess little muscle, the P wave is small. The P wave is best seen in leads II and VI where it is normally a positive deflection. Its shape is rounded and smooth and is less than 0.12 second in duration (see Figure 10.2).
- The PR interval represents the time it takes for the impulse to travel from the SA node to the AV node and the bundle of His and cause ventricular contraction, normally 0.12–0.20 seconds (see Table 10.1).
- The QRS complex represents the spread of impulses by the ventricles. The R wave is the first upward deflection after the P wave. The height of the R wave is variable in different leads but the normal QRS width should be less than 0.12 second or three little squares.

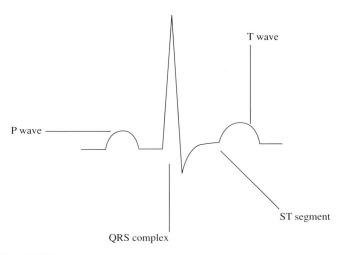

Figure 10.2 The PQRST waves of a sinus rhythm complex.

Table 10.1 Normal PQRST intervals (Jevon 2003, Meek & Morris 2002b).

Interval	Duration	Measurement	Abnormality
PR interval	0.12–0.20 s	From the start of the P wave to the first deflection of QRS	If prolonged, consider delayed or abnormal conduction
QRS interval	0.08–0.12 s	Begins at the Q wave and ends with the S wave deflection	If QRS is >0.12 s consider abnormalities in conduction such as bundle branch block or ventricular arrhythmia. A QRS complex that is <0.12 s will be narrow in shape and originate above the ventricles
QT interval	0.35–0.45 s	From the beginning of QRS until the end of the T wave	Prolonged QT interval is due to hypothermia, drugs and electrolyte disorders such as calcium; may need to be adjusted for age and gender

- The ST segment usually runs fairly flat along the isoelectric line. It signifies the end of ventricular depolarisation and the start of electrical recovery. A rise of 1 mm in either standard or limb leads or a 2-mm rise in the precordial leads is associated with ischaemia or infarction.
- The T wave confirms that repolarisation has taken place. The T wave should be upright in I, II, AVF, V3–V6, inverted in AVR as well as leads III and VI and variable in the remaining leads. The shape of the T wave is usually smooth and rounded.

SHOCKABLE RHYTHMS

Ventricular tachycardia

Ventricular tachycardia (VT) is confirmed by five or more ventricular ectopics in succession and is usually accompanied by a sudden onset of signs and symptoms. VT is normally triggered by an irritable site within the ventricles or macro re-entry circuits; conduction takes place across ventricular cells, rather than along the normal specialised conducting pathway, resulting in the broad shape QRS complexes (>0.12 second in duration). As a consequence of an increased ventricular rate, cardiac output will fall and the patient may lose consciousness. If this rhythm occurs post-myocardial infarction, it can degenerate into ventricular fibrillation (VF).

- VT can be self-terminating or 'non-sustained' when it returns to a normal rhythm within 30 seconds.
- In regular or monomorphic VT, the most common form of this arrhythmia, the appearance between beats is the same. This is in contrast to polymorphic VT (see below under torsades de pointes).

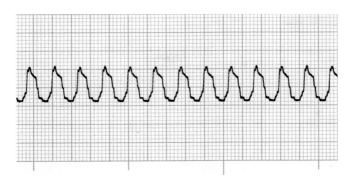

Figure 10.3 Ventricular tachycardia.

Causes
- Ischaemic heart disease (IHD) and myocardial infarction.
- Hypoxia.
- Electrolyte disturbances.
- Drug toxicity or stimulants such as caffeine, nicotine, alcohol.
- Mechanical stimulation from pacing wire or invasive line.

Characteristic features of the ECG (Figure 10.3)
- P wave may be present in some leads and not in others.
- QRS rate between 150 and 300 per minute.
- QRS rhythm may be regular or almost regular, unless fusion beats present.
- QRS broad and wide (>0.12 second or longer).
- Presence of AV dissociation (Edhouse & Morris 2002a).
- There is concordance across the chest leads, meaning that all QRS complexes are either positively or negatively orientated.

Clinical features
Most patients will present with symptoms associated with coronary artery disease or haemodynamic instability due to poor tissue perfusion. Symptoms may include palpitations, chest pain, hypotension, profuse sweating, reduced cognitive functioning and anxiety. The patient may lose consciousness due to a reduced cardiac output.

Response
- Stable patients should be treated with oxygen, have venous access established, and oxygen saturation and baseline observations recorded regularly. Additionally, underlying causes should be identified and treated. A 12-lead ECG should help confirm whether the rhythm is a broad-complex tachycardia (>0.12 second) or whether it is regular or irregular. Treatment will include intravenous amiodarone 300 mg over 20–60 minutes, followed by an infusion of 900 mg over 24 hours. Use of adult tachycardia algorithm (Figure 10.9) helps to tailor further management (Deakin *et al.* 2006).

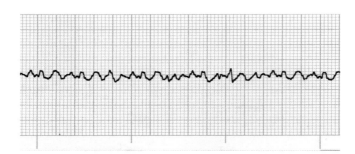

Figure 10.4 Ventricular fibrillation.

- If the patient is unresponsive and cardiac arrest has been confirmed (pulseless VT), follow the treatment outlined in advanced life support (ALS) algorithm (see also Chapter 7).

Ventricular fibrillation

VF is often referred to as chaotic and uncoordinated electrical activity; it is triggered by thousands of ventricular foci discharging at different and rapid rates (shown in Figure 10.4). The lack of strong and regular ventricular contractions causes circulatory collapse and eventually loss of consciousness.

Causes
- Myocardial ischaemia (may occur after myocardial infarction or be associated with a prolonged QT interval).
- Electrolyte disorders such as potassium.
- Cardiomyopathy.
- Accidental electrical shock.
- Digoxin toxicity.
- Hypothermia.

Clinical features
The patient will experience a loss of consciousness, become pulseless and cease breathing.

Characteristic features of the ECG
- P wave and PR interval are unrecognisable.
- QRS rate and rhythm are not definable.
- QRS complex is not discernible.
- There is a wavy line composed of different waves whose amplitude and appearance are variable.
- In the early stages of VF the appearance is coarse but after some minutes it becomes progressively smaller or 'fine VF'. Fine VF can resemble asystole; to distinguish this, increase the gain on the monitor or review the rhythm in a different lead.

Response
- Confirm arrest, summon help and begin external chest compressions and ventilation breaths at a ratio of 30:2 until a defibrillator arrives.
- If a defibrillator is available, apply paddles or self-adhesive pads to the chest, confirm diagnosis of VF, charge the defibrillator and deliver one initial shock (150–200 J biphasic or 360 J monophasic) (European Resuscitation Council (ERC) 2005).
- Follow ALS cardiac arrest algorithm (refer to Chapter 7 for further details).

NON-SHOCKABLE RHYTHMS
Asystole and pulseless electrical activity (PEA) present as clinical emergencies as they are both life-threatening rhythms. The outcome for these non-shockable rhythms is poor unless the underlying factors, which are reversible, can be identified and treated promptly and effectively.

Asystole
Asystole is characterised by complete absence of electrical activity within the heart (see Figure 10.5). According to Gwinnutt *et al.* (2000), asystole is present in 25% of in-hospital cardiac arrests.

Causes
- Extensive coronary artery ischaemia.
- Myocardial infarction.
- Hypoxia.
- Electrolyte imbalance.
- Drug toxicity.
- Prolonged episode of VF.

Clinical features
The patient will suffer a cardiac arrest, become unconscious, cease breathing and no pulse will be palpable.

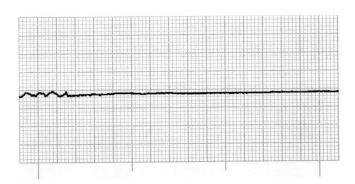

Figure 10.5 Asystole.

Characteristic features of the ECG

- No ECG waveform is recognisable so there is no sign of a rate or a rhythm.
- If only the P waves are present, the rhythm is described as ventricular standstill.
- A flat baseline or trace may appear (this must be differentiated from fine VF). Asystole must be established by reviewing the leads and checking they are attached to the patient, increasing the gain and comparing the rhythm through two different leads (Jevon 2003).
- Spurious asystole (after multiple defibrillations) must be excluded; use ECG leads for monitoring.

Response

- If the patient is unresponsive, start CPR at 30:2.
- When monitor or defibrillator is available, confirm that rhythm in asystole; without stopping CPR, check that leads are correctly attached.
- Check ECG for evidence of a P wave, as this may respond well to cardiac pacing (Deakin *et al.* 2006).
- Follow right-sided path of ALS algorithm (see Chapter 7).

Pulseless electrical activity

In PEA, electrical activity in the form of regular or near-regular complexes can be observed on a cardiac monitor, although palpable arterial pulses are absent. Data from Gwinnutt *et al.* (2000) suggest that PEA features in approximately 35% of all in-hospital arrests, although this figure might be higher. Survival after cardiac arrest from either asystole or PEA is poor; however, the latter usually linked with non-coronary aetiologies. Success depends on whether the underlying cause is reversible and treated efficiently. There are two forms of PEA, primary and secondary (Jevon 2003).

- Primary PEA – brought on by myocardial fibres not contracting effectively, resulting in the loss of cardiac output. It can be associated with large MI, drugs, calcium-channel blockers, poisoning and electrolyte disturbances including hyperkalaemia and hypocalcaemia.
- Secondary PEA – the result of a mechanical problem that impedes ventricular filling or ejection. The causes include pulmonary embolism, ventricular wall rupture, tension pneumothorax, aortic dissection or rupture, hypovolaemia and cardiac tamponade. Pulmonary embolism is a common cause of PEA in both in-hospital and out-of-hospital arrests (Virkkunen *et al.* 2008).

Clinical features

- Absence of palpable pulses.
- Physical signs of a cardiac arrest.

Characteristic features of the ECG

- ECG monitor displays electrical activity in the form of a regular or irregular rhythm.

- Atrial fibrillation (AF) is commonly associated in patients presenting with PEA.

Response
- Confirm that patient has arrested and start CPR 30:2. Confirm that ECG leads are attached correctly.
- Administer adrenaline 1 mg once intravenous access is established.
- Continue treatment as outlined in the ALS algorithm (see Chapter 7).
- Identify and treat reversible causes, e.g. the four H's and the four T's (see Chapter 13).

PERI-ARREST ARRHYTHMIAS

Peri-arrest rhythms are those that may present as emergency situations. Many of these adverse arrhythmias may precede VF or occur after myocardial infarction or successful defibrillation. In initial instances, if standard measures for use by non-specialists fail to prevent or correct arrhythmias, consultation with experts must be sought (ERC 2005).

Key principles of treatment
- Administer oxygen.
- Establish venous access.
- Obtain a 12-lead ECG.
- Assess for and correct any electrolyte disturbances (e.g. magnesium, potassium or calcium).

The aim of assessment and treatment is twofold:

(a) establish the patient's condition – stable or unstable;
(b) identify the underlying rhythm disturbance.

Recognising adverse signs
Assessment and management strategies should be directed at establishing the clinical status of the patient, and the origin and character of the arrhythmia. Adverse arrhythmias can manifest with the following:

- Evidence of a low cardiac output – for example, hypotension (systolic blood pressure of <90 mm Hg), cool peripheries, clamminess, pallor and confusion.
- Excessive tachycardia – a narrow- or broad-complex tachycardia can significantly decrease diastolic time, resulting in impaired coronary blood flow and lead to myocardial ischaemia.
- Excessive bradycardia – usually defined as a rate less than 40 bpm, although some patients with low cardiac reserve may become symptomatic at rates of 60 bpm.
- Heart failure – in acute episodes, an arrhythmia may compromise myocardial performance and patients may present with pulmonary oedema, a raised jugular venous pressure and hepatic engorgement – typical of right-sided heart failure

- Chest pain can be precipitated by an arrhythmia, most commonly a tachycardia, as a manifestation of coronary ischaemia. The consequences may be more serious if the patient has a history of coronary heart disease (Deakin *et al.* 2006).

Treatment options

Three main options are available (ERC 2005):

- pharmacological therapies – anti-arrhythmic drugs tend to be less predictable and act much slower than electrical cardioversion in restoring sinus rhythm. More suitable for clinical stable patients;
- electrical cardioversion is recommended for patients presenting adverse clinical signs;
- cardiac pacing.

The major peri-arrest rhythms include:

- bradycardia;
- atrial fibrillation;
- other narrow-complex tachycardia;
- broad-complex tachycardia.

Bradycardia

A heart rate of less than 60 bpm is used to describe a bradycardic rhythm, although there are many healthy individuals, such as athletes, who are clinically well despite having a slow heart rate (Da Costa *et al.* 2002). Recent classifications describe 'absolute' bradycardia when rate is less than 40 per minute and when the heart rate is inappropriately slow to sustain haemodynamic functioning, this is termed 'relative' (Deakin *et al.* 2006).

Bradycardias (see Figure 10.6) may occur due to cardiac or non-cardiac disorders and the following signs may be indicative of instability:

- a systolic blood pressure <90 mm Hg;
- a pulse rate of <40 per minute;
- ventricular arrhythmias needing suppression;
- heart failure.

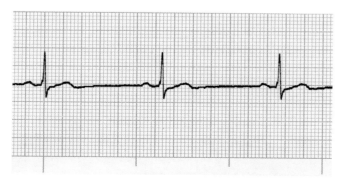

Figure 10.6 Bradycardia

Causes
- Hypothermia.
- Drugs (beta-blockers, some calcium-channel blockers, digoxin).
- Hypothyroidism.
- Sick sinus syndrome.
- Electrolyte disorders.
- Patients with inferior myocardial infarctions are prone to suffer from a bradycardic episode, due to the involvement of the right coronary artery.

Characteristic features of the ECG
These depend on the underlying rhythm:

- slow heart rates;
- P waves may appear regularly or intermittently;
- variable regular or irregular ventricular rates.

Response
If signs of deterioration are present:

- administer atropine 500 µg via an intravenous access;
- the dose may be repeated every 3–5 minutes to a maximum of 3 mg (see Figure 10.7).

If there is a positive response to atropine or if the patient is stable, the risk of asystole must be ascertained – this may be present if there is:

- a recent history of asystole;
- Mobitz type II AV block;
- ventricular standstill greater than 3 seconds;
- complete heart block with a wide QRS (as seen in Figure 10.8).

For patients who have failed to respond to atropine or are unstable, transvenous pacing is necessary. If pacing facilities are not immediately available, the following can be employed as temporary measures:

- transcutaneous pacing;
- titrate low-dose adrenaline infusion in the range 2–10 µg/min.

Dopamine, isoprenaline and theophylline may be used for patients with symptoms precipitated by bradycardia. If it is suspected that the cause of bradycardia may be due to beta-blockers or calcium-channel blockers, these drugs must be stopped and intravenous glucagon should be given (Deakin *et al.* 2006).

Tachycardias

As the treatment principles for broad-complex tachycardia, narrow-complex tachycardia and AF are similar to all, they have been consolidated into one single adult (with pulse) tachycardia algorithm (Figure 10.9). The management of a tachycardia will be guided by whether it is unstable as indicated by signs of impaired cognitive status, hypotension, chest pain, heart failure and other signs of

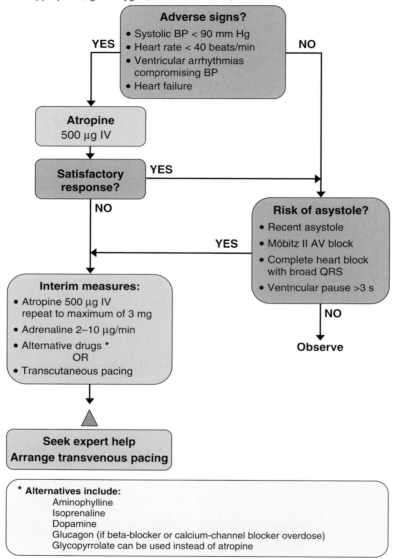

Adult bradycardia algorithm
(includes rates inappropriately slow for haemodynamic state)

If appropriate, give oxygen, cannulate a vein, and record a 12-lead ECG

Adverse signs?
- Systolic BP < 90 mm Hg
- Heart rate < 40 beats/min
- Ventricular arrhythmias compromising BP
- Heart failure

YES → **Atropine** 500 μg IV → **Satisfactory response?**

NO (from Adverse signs?) and YES (from Satisfactory response?) →

Risk of asystole?
- Recent asystole
- Möbitz II AV block
- Complete heart block with broad QRS
- Ventricular pause >3 s

YES →

Interim measures:
- Atropine 500 μg IV repeat to maximum of 3 mg
- Adrenaline 2–10 μg/min
- Alternative drugs *
  OR
- Transcutaneous pacing

NO → **Observe**

↓

Seek expert help
Arrange transvenous pacing

---

* **Alternatives include:**
Aminophylline
Isoprenaline
Dopamine
Glucagon (if beta-blocker or calcium-channel blocker overdose)
Glycopyrrolate can be used instead of atropine

Figure 10.7 Bradycardia algorithm. (*Source*: Resuscitation Council UK, Resuscitation Guidelines 2005. Reproduced with kind permission of the Resuscitation Council UK.)

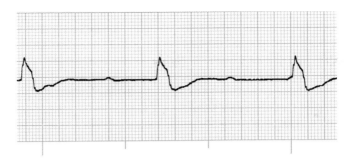

Figure 10.8 Complete heart block.

shock. For these patients immediate electrical synchronised cardioversion should be performed.

For both broad-complex tachycardias and AF cardioversion should start with 120–150 J shock for biphasic defibrillators (200 J for monophasic defibrillators). If the arrhythmia persists, energy levels should be increased incrementally. By contrast, atrial flutter and narrow-complex tachycardias respond better to lower energies. It is recommended to begin with 70–120 J if using a biphasic defibrillator or 100 J for a monophasic defibrillator (ERC 2005).

Should cardioversion fail to reinstate sinus rhythm and the patient remain haemodynamically compromised, a loading dose of intravenous amiodarone 300 mg should be administered over 10–20 minutes followed by a further attempt at electrical cardioversion. The initial dose of amiodarone may be followed by 900 mg infused over 24 hours (see Figure 10.9).

Stable patients, presenting without adverse signs or symptoms triggered by the arrhythmia, and not deteriorating, should have their ECG trace carefully reviewed to determine whether it is a narrow-complex or broad-complex tachycardia. Referral to experts is recommended to establish the range of treatment options available. If the patient becomes unstable due to a tachyarrhythmia, then immediate synchronised electrical cardioversion should be performed. If a tachyarrhythmia is precipitated as a result of a co-morbid illness, treatment of underlying condition is also essential.

Broad-complex tachycardias

These are associated with a QRS >0.12 second in duration and usually originate within the ventricles; however, they may be triggered by a supraventricular rhythms with aberrant conduction.

In the situation where a patient is clinically unstable, it should be assumed that the rhythm is ventricular in origin and electrical cardioversion should be attempted followed by the intravenous administration of amiodarone (see Figure 10.9). Should a patient with a broad-complex tachycardia be clinically stable, confirming whether the rhythm is regular or irregular is the next step (Deakin *et al.* 2006).

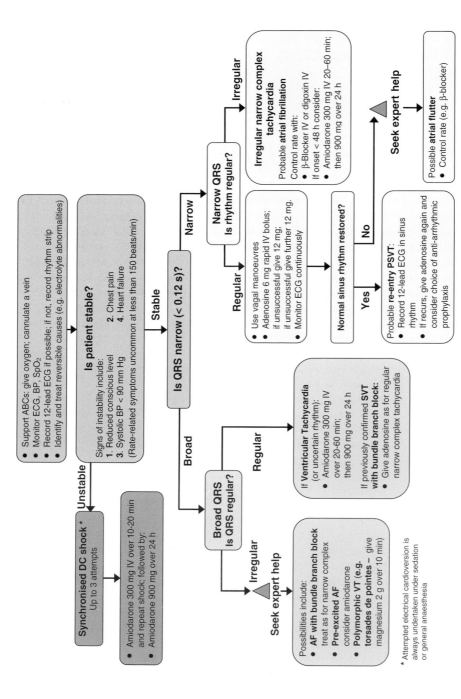

Figure 10.9 Adult tachycardia algorithm (with pulse). (*Source*: Resuscitation Council UK, Resuscitation Guidelines 2005. Reproduced with kind permission of the Resuscitation Council UK.)

Regular broad-complex tachycardia

This is most likely to be VT or supraventricular tachycardia with bundle branch block. Patients without adverse signs should be treated with a loading dose of amioderone followed by maintenance infusion (see Figure 10.9). Stable patients with a broad-complex tachycardia, which is known to be supraventricular tachycardia with bundle branch block, should be given adenosine as recommended for narrow-complex tachycardia (ERC 2005).

Irregular broad-complex tachycardia

This is most likely to manifest as AF with bundle branch block, but review of 12-lead ECG by a clinical expert will confirm this. These patients should be managed as for AF, see below. Clinicians should also consider AF with ventricular excitation (common among patients with Wolff-Parkinson-White (WPW) syndrome) or polymorphic VT (see below), as causes for irregular broad-complex tachycardia. Patients with pre-excited AF or atrial flutter respond well to synchronised cardioversion. Patients presenting with the polymorphic VT or torsades de pointes are unlikely to be stable (ERC 2005).

Torsades de pointes is an irregular broad-complex tachycardia or polymorphic VT. Here, there is a wide beat-to-beat variation in the QRS morphology rotating every 5–20 per minute along the baseline (Spearritt 2003). Torsades de pointes represents an uncommon variant form of VT which may deteriorate into VF. It may occur after a myocardial infarction or be associated with prolonged repolarisation known as QT syndromes. IHD, hypomagnesaemia, antiarrhythmics, antibacterials and bradycardia due to sick sinus syndrome precipitate torsades de pointes (Edhouse & Morris 2002b). Treatment involves stopping any drug that prolongs the QT interval, correcting electrolyte imbalances such as potassium. Treatment may include the administration of intravenous magnesium sulphate, 2 mg over 10 minutes (refer to Figure 10.9). If unsuccessful, overdrive pacing may be required once the arrhythmia has stabilised (Deakin *et al.* 2006). However, if the patient displays signs of deterioration and pulses become absent, immediate defibrillation should be performed (follow ALS algorithm, Chapter 7).

Narrow-complex tachycardias

These include rhythms with a QRS complex of <0.12 second and are also divided into regular and irregular narrow-complex tachycardias

Regular narrow-complex tachycardia

This includes the following:

- sinus tachycardia;
- AV nodal re-entry tachycardia (AVRNT) – most common form of regular narrow-complex tachycardia;
- AV re-entry tachycardia (AVRT), associated with WPW syndrome;
- atrial flutter with regular atrioventricular conduction (normally 2:1).

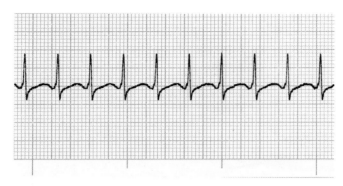

Figure 10.10 A narrow-complex tachycardia.

Sinus tachycardia

Heart rates may increase due to exercise, or anxiety, as part of normal physiological response. In ill-health, other stimuli such as pain or blood loss and medications may produce a similar effect. Identifying the underlying cause should inform subsequent treatments.

AVRNT and AVRT (paroxysmal supraventricular tachycardia)

AVRNT is the most usual form of paroxysmal supraventricular tachycardia, often presenting in patients without any history of heart disease. Patients may experience symptoms which could be disturbing and the reason for seeking help. ECG characteristic features (see Figure 10.10) may include:

- P waves are not always detectable;
- PR interval is not measurable;
- the relationship between P waves and QRS complex is not discernible;
- there is a QRS rate of 150–250 per minute;
- QRS rate tends to be regular;
- QRS complex tends to be narrow (<0.12 second), unlike VT;
- the V leads are discordant (some are positive and others negative) on examination of the 12-lead ECG.

Patients most likely to experience AVRT have WPW syndrome. In the absence of any structural heart disease, the rhythm is, as above, likely to be benign.

Atrial flutter with regular AV conduction

This produces a regular and narrow-complex tachycardia, but determining atrial activity or the presence of flutter waves can be difficult. Differentiating this rhythm in the presence of AVRNT and AVRT may require advice from experts. Atrial flutter with 2:1 block will result in a tachycardia of 150 bpm, assuming a flutter rate of 300 bpm.

Response

Where a patient display adverse signs, which are provoked by an arrhythmia, the individual must be sedated and synchronised cardioversion administered. These patients may also be treated with adenosine while waiting for cardioversion facilities to be ready. If adenosine does not restore sinus rhythm, electrical cardioversion should not be deferred (Deakin *et al.* 2006). In the absence of contraindications and the patient is stable, the following should be considered:

- Vagal manoeuvres (carotid sinus massage or the valsalva manoeuvre) will stop up to a quarter of paroxysmal SVT episodes; a 12-lead ECG tracing should be recorded with each procedure.
- For carotid sinus massage, the pulse has to be located and then massaged. If there is evidence of a carotid bruit this technique should be avoided due to possible complications; inexperienced personnel should not perform carotid sinus massage. Bradycardia is another side effect of this technique which may degenerate into VF; therefore, recording an ECG during each procedure is advised.
- The valsalva manoeuvre involves asking the patient to cough or to blow into a 20-mL syringe, inducing a strain effect which forces expiration against a closed glottis. A valsalva manoeuvre is most successful if the casualty is placed supine.
- If vagal stimulants fail and atrial flutter is not present, intravenous adenosine 6 mg may be administered rapidly in a bolus and flushed with saline. If unsuccessful, a dose of 12 mg can be given and repeated if the rhythm persists. An ECG trace should be obtained during each injection. The effect of adenosine is to inhibit or slow conduction of impulses across the AV node. The patient should be warned that they might feel unpleasant sensations in the chest.
- Vagal manoeuvres or adenosine should be effective in immediately terminating AVNRT or AVRT. A non-termination of regular narrow-complex tachycardia with adenosine is indicative of atrial tachycardia, for example atrial flutter.
- If vagal manoeuvres or adenosine fail to stop regular narrow-complex tachycardia, calcium-channel blockers, such as verapamil 2.5–5 mg can be considered (Deakin *et al.* 2006, ERC 2005).
- Irregular narrow-complex tachycardia.

Commonly this is likely to be AF (see Figure 10.11) and more unusually atrial flutter with variable block. A 12-lead ECG trace will help to accurately identify the rhythm. If as a result of the arrhythmia, a patient becomes clinically unstable, synchronised electrical cardioversion should be attempted.

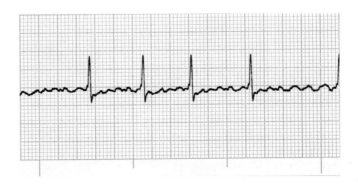

Figure 10.11 Atrial fibrillation.

If no other signs of deterioration are evident, treatment alternatives include (Deakin *et al.* 2006):

- rate control by drug therapy;
- rhythm control by conversion to sinus rhythm using pharmacological measures;
- rhythm control by electrical cardioversion;
- maintenance of sinus rhythm and prevention of complications (e.g. thromboembolic events).

Patients who have been in AF for more than 48 hours should be anticoagulated for at least three weeks, or absence of atrial thrombus has been confirmed by trans-oesophageal echcocardiography, before cardioversion either chemically or electrically is considered. If rate control is necessary, this may be achieved with beta-blockers, digoxin, magnesium or a combination of these (Resuscitation Council UK 2005). Conversely, if AF has been present for less than 48 hours in duration, rhythm control may be achieved with amioderone (see Figure 10.8).

Synchronised cardioversion is an alternative option and more effective in returning the majority of patients to sinus rhythm when compared to chemical therapies. Biphasic waveforms are more effective in treating AF than monophasic waveforms for cardioversion, therefore use the former in preference (Deakin & Nolan 2005). When either AF is unknown or in the case of ventricular pre-excitation, expert advice should be sought. Recent guidelines for the management of patients with AF have been published by the American College of Cardiology, the American Heart Association and the European Society of Cardiology (2006).

REVIEW OF LEARNING

- ❏ To be able to *recognise* and *respond* to potential and actual life-threatening arrhythmias, an understanding of the basic conduction system and the characteristics of sinus rhythm is essential.
- ❏ Prior to attaching the leads to the monitor, check that all equipment is in good working order and within date of expiry.
- ❏ Cardiac monitors, defibrillator paddles and AED adhesive electrodes should be used to assess the underlying heart rhythm. Interruption of CPR should be kept to a minimum.
- ❏ Shockable rhythms include VF and pulseless VT.
- ❏ If the patient presents in asystole, it is important to check that all the leads are correctly connected, and the gain increased to eliminate the possibility of fine VF.
- ❏ Healthcare professionals must be suspicious of the patient who presents with absent pulses but whose ECG monitor displays signs of electrical activity.
- ❏ Peri-arrest arrhythmias pose a risk to patients. Knowledge of these rhythms and treatment algorithms enhance the effectiveness of the healthcare professional. Expert advice from cardiologists may be required to accurately interpret underlying mechanisms for some of the more complex tachycardias.
- ❏ The ALS algorithm for the management of the adult in cardiac arrest provides guidance on treatment actions.

Case study

Mrs Wilson is a 67-year-old woman who arrives at your ward with a history of chest pain and episodes of feeling faint. After some formalities, you explain that you need to attach her to the monitor to obtain a continuous display of her heart rhythm. Mrs Wilson consents to the procedure and you draw the curtains.

How do you make certain that the ECG display on the monitor screen is of high quality?

Prior to starting, inspect the leads and the cable connected to the monitor, check for signs of damage and, if soiled, clean before use. Check electrodes to make sure that they are in date and intact, then attach according to local practice. Ensure a good contact with the patient's skin. To avoid interference, make certain that the electrodes are placed over bone, and to obtain good contact, make sure that the skin is dry.

Place the ECG electrodes away from areas that could be used for defibrillation. If there is a poor signal, replace the electrodes and check all connections as well as the lead for signs of damage. If the patient becomes clammy, change the electrodes more frequently. Should the complexes appear too small, check the patient, select another lead and increase the amplitude or replace electrodes. Finally, set the alarms and explain to the patient their significance and factors which may inadvertently set them off.

You note that Mrs Wilson's rhythm appears regular and the digital display indicates that her rate is 90 bpm. Discuss the features of: P, QRS, ST and T waves. For a complete answer, review the appropriate section of the chapter.

Whilst you are taking the history, Mrs Wilson complains of increasing chest pain. You reassure her and administer oxygen via mask. Whilst doing this you are aware that the non-invasive blood pressure has fallen to 90/60 mm Hg, she has a tachycardia of more than 150 bpm and has become clammy.

Discuss the symptoms and ECG characteristics of VT.

In VT, the patient may or may not be responsive. In addition, the ECG will reveal key changes which can be found earlier in this chapter.

CONCLUSION

The ECG is a diagnostic tool used to assess cardiac rhythms continuously and provide an indication of changes within the heart's function. To be of value, healthcare staff must ensure that they are familiar with the techniques for ensuring that a high-quality ECG trace is displayed on the screen and know how to minimise artefacts and sources of interference. Being able to recognise shockable, non-shockable and peri-arrest rhythms and how to respond to these emergency situations also requires practice supported by undertaking additional educational input.

REFERENCES

American College of Cardiology, American Heart Association & the European Cardiac Society (2006) Guidelines for the management of patients with atrial fibrillation. *Europace* **8**, 651–745.

Da Costa, D., Brady, W.J. & Edhouse, J. (2002) ABC of clinical electrocardiography: bradycardias and atrioventricular conduction block. *British Medical Journal* **324**, 535–8.

Deakin, C.D. & Nolan, J. (2005) European Resuscitation Council guidelines for resuscitation 2005. Section 3: Electrical therapies: automated external defibrillators, defibrillation, cardioversion and pacing. *Resuscitation* **67** (suppl 1), S25–37.

Deakin, C.D., Nolan, J.P., Soar, J., Bottinger, B.W. & Smith, G. (2006) Advanced life support. In: Baskett, P. & Nolan, J. (eds) *A Pocket Book of the European Resuscitation Council Guidelines for Resuscitation 2005*. Elsevier, London.

Edhouse, J. & Morris, F. (2002a) ABC of clinical electrocardiography: broad complex tachycardia – Part I. *British Medical Journal* **324**, 719–22.

Edhouse, J. & Morris, F. (2002b) ABC of clinical electrocardiography: broad complex tachycardia – Part II. *British Medical Journal* **324**, 776–9.

European Resuscitation Council (2005) European Resuscitation Council guidelines for resuscitation 2005. Section 4: adult advanced life support. *Resuscitation* **67** (suppl 1), S39–86.

Gwinnutt, C., Coulumbo, M. & Harris, R. (2000) Outcome after cardiac arrest in adults in UK hospitals: effect of the 1997 guidelines. *Resuscitation* **47**, 125–35.

Jevon, P. (2003) *ECGs for Nurses*. Blackwell Publishing, Oxford.

Meek, S. & Morris, F. (2002a) Introduction I – leads, rate, rhythm and cardiac axis. *British Medical Journal* **324**, 415–18.

Meek, S. & Morris, F. (2002b) Introduction II – basic terminology. *British Medical Journal* **324**, 470–73.

Spearritt, D. (2003) Torsades de pointes following cardioversion: case history and literature review. *Australian Critical Care* **16** (4), 144–9.

Virkkunen, I., Paaiso, L., Ryynänen, S. *et al.* (2008) Pulseless electrical activity and unsuccessful out-of-hospital resuscitation: what is the cause of death? *Resuscitation* **7**, 210–10.

Defibrillation Theory and Practice

11

John W. Albarran & Pam Moule

INTRODUCTION

Survival outcomes after a cardiac arrest depend on recognising the victim and responding with early defibrillation. Defibrillation is a major link in the Chain of Survival (see Chapter 5) and remains one of the most clinically effective interventions for improving outcomes following ventricular fibrillation (VF) and pulseless ventricular tachycardia (VT) arrest. Traditionally, the skill of defibrillation has been confined to those working in critical care areas, but due to advances in technology other healthcare professionals can learn how to defibrillate safely and effectively. Indeed, the introduction of smaller, lighter and easier to operate automated external defibrillators (AEDs) that are highly sensitive and reliable enables the cardiac rhythm to be assessed without delaying the initiation or interrupting progress of cardiopulmonary resuscitation (CPR).

In response to the effectiveness of early defibrillation in reducing mortality rates from VT/VF, the American Heart Association in collaboration with the International Liaison Committee on Resuscitation (AHA and ILCOR 2000) issued guidelines for training in AED use to be part of basic life support (BLS). The guidelines have been informed by the past three decades of research which have demonstrated that AEDs could be safely and appropriately used by a number of healthcare providers, first providers and lay people (Moule & Albarran 2002). Confidence in the ability of lay people and other rescuers to operate AEDs following minimal training resulted in recommendations by the European Resuscitation Council (ERC) (Bossaert *et al*. 1998) and the Resuscitation Council UK (2000) that all healthcare staff who may need to respond to a cardiopulmonary emergency must be competent in BLS and be authorised to perform defibrillation using an AED.

AIMS

This chapter introduces the current concepts of defibrillation and synchronised cardioversion based on the most recent recommendations issued by the European Resuscitation Council (Deakin & Nolan 2005) and provides standardised guidance on how to operate a defibrillator safely and effectively.

LEARNING OUTCOMES

By the end of the chapter, the reader will be able to:

❏ discuss the *basic principles and purpose of early defibrillation*;
❏ discuss the *factors that impact on successful defibrillation*;
❏ describe the key components in *operating a manual defibrillator*;
❏ explain the principles and procedures associated with *synchronised cardioversion*;
❏ demonstrate knowledge of the *broad safety issues* when operating a defibrillator;
❏ describe the roles and functions of *implantable cardiac defibrillators*.

PRINCIPLES AND PURPOSE OF EARLY DEFIBRILLATION

According to Gwinnutt *et al.* (2000) and Holmberg *et al.* (2000), VF and VT are the initial presenting rhythms in about 30% of in-hospital cardiac arrests and in around 85% out-of-hospital cardiac arrests.

Patients with myocardial ischaemia or an infarction are most likely to experience an episode of VF or VT, which may be exacerbated by stress and cardiac pain. The release of circulating catecholamines, part of a primitive response, can increase the heart rate and myocardial workload and precipitate ventricular ectopics. The ectopics may eventually convert into VF or VT. For those who develop these rhythms, the loss of a regular cardiac output will accelerate myocardial ischaemia, metabolic acidosis, tissue hypoxia, acute under-perfusion of vital organs and sudden death.

Defibrillation aims to deliver an electrical current of sufficient magnitude across the myocardium to depolarise a critical mass of myocardium in order to restore coordinated electrical and mechanical activity (Deakin & Nolan 2005). Post-shock myocardial cells enter a period of recovery, reset themselves and allow the sinoatrial node to restore sinus rhythm activity and produce organised myocardial fibre contraction (Cooper *et al.* 1998, Harris 2002). The absence of VF/VT at five seconds after shock delivery and the return of spontaneous circulation more accurately define the goals of defibrillation. However, there are factors that may influence the outcomes of in-hospital resuscitation (as shown in Box 11.1). In particular, the provision of quality chest compressions prior to defibrillation may be associated with better survival outcomes for cardiac arrest due to defibrillation (Cobbe *et al.* 1991, Endelson *et al.* 2006, Wik *et al.* 2003). A number of theories have been postulated; however, changes in the behaviour of the ventricles seem pertinent (Chamberlain *et al.* 2008).

Arrhythmias may also be triggered as a result of:

- *Cardiac disorders* – hypoxia, hypothermia, electrolyte disorders, drug toxicity (digoxin), electrocution and any cause leading to hypoxaemia.
- *Airway obstruction* – laryngospasm, foreign bodies, vomit and loss of airway control as a result of damage to central nervous system (CNS).
- *Respiratory failure* – pulmonary oedema, acute asthma, decreased respiratory drive due to CNS changes and inadequate respiratory effort as a result of exhaustion or opioid abuse.

Box 11.1   Factors affecting outcomes of in-hospital resuscitation.

There are a number of factors that have a bearing on successful in-hospital resuscitation.

- **Early recognition of VT and VF** – improved outcomes occur if staff trained to defibrillate use an AED within three minutes or sooner after the arrest has been confirmed and before the arrival of the arrest team.
- **The provision of CPR prior to defibrillation** – the delivery of quality CPR prior to the administration of a defibrillator shock is associated with increased survival following cardiac arrest (Cobb *et al.* 1999, Endelson *et al.* 2006, Wik *et al.* 2003).
- **Time taken to deliver a shock** – statistics indicate that for every minute that elapses before defibrillation, between 7 and 10% of patients will die who might have otherwise been saved (Cobbe *et al.* 1991, Valenzuela *et al.* 2000).
- **Patient variables** – if the patient is less than 70 years of age and a return of spontaneous circulation occurs within three minutes or less, then survival from cardiac arrest is more likely.
- **Location of the arrest** – in the past patients in general wards experienced reduced survival outcomes following a cardiac arrest; however, this trend is likely to end with increased training and competence in AED use (Coady 1999, Soar & Mckay 1998, Spearpoint *et al.* 2000).

STRATEGIES FOR SAFE DEFIBRILLATION

Pre-defibrillation strategies

Safe use of oxygen

In the presence of oxygen, sparking leading to burns of a patient's skin can be the result of poorly applied defibrillator paddles. The following are suggested strategies to overcome this risk during defibrillation:

- Remove oxygen mask or nasal cannulae and place at least 1 m away from the patient.
- If a ventilation bag or other airway adjunct is attached to a tracheal tube leave connected to the patient. Alternatively, prior to attempted defibrillation disconnect the ventilation bag from tracheal tube and place it at least 1 m from the patient's chest.
- If the patient is attached to a mechanical ventilator, ventilator tubing circuit should be left connected to the tracheal tube. It may be appropriate for therapeutic reasons to leave the patient connected to the ventilator during shock delivery. Should disconnection from ventilator be necessary, the machine should be switched off and oxygen delivered by ventilation bag. During defibrillation, remove ventilation circuit and oxygen supply to 1 m away from the patient's chest (Deakin & Nolan 2005). The use of self-adhesive pads is safer as it reduces the risk of sparks.

Transthoracic impedance (TTI) plays a part in the level of cardiac response to a defibrillatory shock. TTI is defined as the resistance to current flow through chest wall, lung tissue and myocardium; hence, the greater the resistance, the less the flow of current (Cooper *et al.* 1998). There are a number of practical means by which TTI can be reduced.

Shaving the chest

A hairy chest can cause air trapping below an electrode and poor skin to electrode contact. This results in high TTI, ineffective defibrillation and the risk of arcing (e.g. sparks occurring from electrode to electrode or skin to electrode) which can cause burns on the patient's chest. If equipment is immediately available, the areas intended for electrode placement should be shaved. However, defibrillation should not be delayed if there is no shaving equipment available.

Paddle force

When using handheld paddles, a force of 8 kg in adults and 5 kg for children of 1–8 years should be applied (see Figure 11.1). Firm paddle pressure decreases

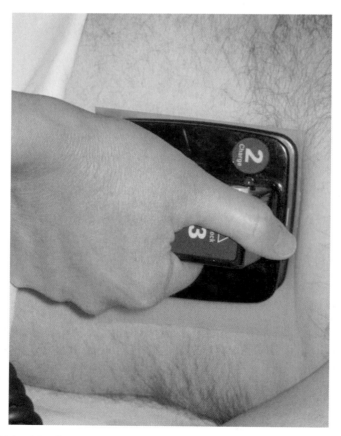

Figure 11.1 Maintaining firm paddle pressure.

TTI by improving contact between paddle and skin surface lessening thoracic volume. Since paddles have a bare metal surface, there is a risk of arcing, high TTI and superficial cutaneous burns; however, these adverse effects can be minimised and electrical conduction improved by using gel pads (Deakin *et al.* 2006). Electrode pastes should be avoided as they tend to smear and increase the chance of superficial dermal burns and ineffective defibrillation.

Electrode position

Positioning of electrodes (pads or paddles) is important although its role as a determinant in improving outcomes of either return of spontaneous circulation or survival of VT/VF is not established (Deakin & Nolan 2005). However, many studies have shown that healthcare professionals and lay people have difficulties with accurate placement of electrodes (Moule *et al.* 2008, Whitfield *et al.* 2003).

Current evidence indicates that optimum transmyocardial current during defibrillation happens when the fibrillating heart chambers lie directly between the electrodes. The implications of this are that electrode position for either ventricular or atrial arrhythmias may not be the same; consequently, the following recommendations have been proposed (Deakin *et al.* 2006).

- Electrode placement for ventricular arrhythmias: The right 'sternal' electrode must be placed to the right of the sternum, below the right clavicle. The apical electrode positioned in the mid-axillary line, level with ECG electrode V_6 or female breast (see Figures 11.2 and 11.3). It is important that placement of the apex paddle is suitably lateral and is away from any breast tissue as this helps decrease thoracic impedance and raises current flow.
- Other optional electrode positions:
  - In the bi-axillary approach, electrodes are placed laterally, to the right and left sides of the chest wall.
  - Alternatively, one electrode can be sited in the standard apical position, the other on the right or left upper back.
  - The anterior electrode can also be placed to the left precordium (the sternal border) and the remaining electrode posterior to the heart just below the left scapula. This approach is not easy, particularly if the patient is of large size. It should be used only when defibrillation with standard paddle technique has been ineffective or if the patient has an internal pacemaker or implantable cardiac defibrillator.
- Electrode placement for atrial arrhythmias:
  - The anterior–posterior option is more effective than the conventional antero-apical in the elective cardioversion of atrial fibrillation. This may be less significant when using biphasic waveform defibrillators; however, both are acceptable and safe for the cardioversion of atrial arrhythmias (Deakin & Nolan 2005).

Respiratory phase

During respiration TTI varies, but it is lowest at the end of expiration. Ideally, defibrillation should be attempted at the end of expiration when there is less air in the lungs; thus, reducing the distance between electrodes and heart. In

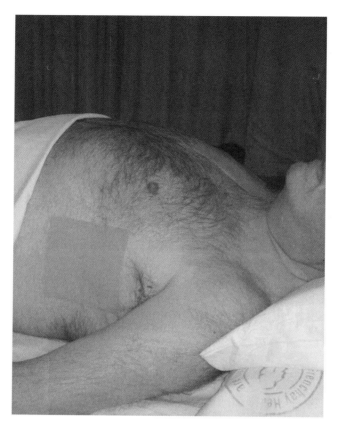

Figure 11.2 Recommended position of apical electrode gel pad.

mechanically ventilated patients, use of positive-end-expiratory pressure (PEEP) will increase TTI; therefore, this should be decreased during defibrillation (Deakin *et al.* 1998).

Electrode size
Typically, large size electrodes have lower impedance but oversized electrodes can produce less across the myocardial current flow (Deakin & Nolan 2005).

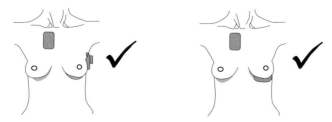

Figure 11.3 Under-breast and lateral-to-breast paddle positions. (Adapted from Pagan-Carlo *et al.* 1996.)

The surface area covered by both electrodes should be at least 150 cm^2. Whether for handheld paddles or self-adhesive gel pads, electrodes of 8–12 cm in diameter are appropriate and effective for use in adults. However, electrodes of 12 cm produce higher defibrillation success than those of 8 cm in diameter.

Pads versus paddles
It is always preferable to use self-adhesive because the risks of arcing are greatly reduced and, unlike manual defibrillators, providers can defibrillate a casualty at a safe distance. Both defibrillation paddles and self-adhesive pads are suitable for quick monitoring of the underlying cardiac rhythm and for providing a rapid first defibrillator shock (Deakin *et al.* 2006).

Energy requirements and waveforms
Due to time delays with a three-shock sequence and interruptions of CPR for rhythm analysis, defibrillation guidelines were revised and updated. Current practice recommends delivering a single defibrillation shock of 150 J (biphasic), or 360 J (monophasic) and resuming CPR at a rate of 30 compressions and two respirations. This sequence should proceed without stopping to assess the cardiac rhythm or feeling for a pulse (refer to Chapter 7). Successful restoration of a perfusing rhythm may not be immediately accompanied by a palpable pulse; therefore, CPR should be continued. The single shock approach applies to biphasic and monophasic defibrillators, although the ideal energy levels for either of the waveforms are unknown and recommendations reflect expert consensus based on a review of the evidence (Deakin & Nolan 2005).

The two most common waveforms are 'monophasic' and 'biphasic', their shape being determined by the flow of electrical current and TTI.

- *Monophasic* waveforms are currents that flow in one direction between electrodes over a specific period and are generated by stored energy being discharged from a capacitor through the chest. Because of their poorer efficacy, when compared to biphasic waveforms, the recommended first shock energy level when using a monophasic defibrillator is 360 J.
- *Biphasic* waveforms provide bidirectional flow of current in two phases at a much lower energy than conventional defibrillators. Initially, the current flows in a positive direction for a specified period and once the first phase is complete, the current then reverses and flows in a negative direction for the same period of the electrical discharge (Faddy *et al.* 2003, Harris 2002, Tang *et al.* 2000).

The advantage of integrating biphasic waveform technology into modern defibrillators is that at lower energies, biphasic defibrillators are more efficacious in terminating VF than standard 200 J monophasic waveforms (Faddy *et al.* 2003, Wanchun *et al.* 2000). The benefits of lower energy levels include:

- early restoration of spontaneous circulation;
- reduced myocardial injury;
- decreased signs of ST segment elevation;
- potential hazards can be reduced.

The recommended first shock energy level for a biphasic defibrillator should be at least 150 J. Ideally, defibrillator designers should incorporate data on waveform dose range; however, if this information is not available, the provider should administer a dose of 200 J for the first shock. This default dose should apply only if devices are not clearly labelled or if the operator is unfamiliar with the defibrillator (Deakin & Nolan 2005).

Second and subsequent shocks:

- Biphasic defibrillators – current recommendations include using initial energy levels of 150–200 J. If the initial shock is ineffective, second and subsequent shocks can be given at 150–360 J.
- Monophasic defibrillators – if initial shock at 360 J is unsuccessful, maintain energy levels for initial and subsequent shocks at 360 J.

OTHER PRACTICAL CONSIDERATIONS

Check casualty

- Transdermal drug patches should be removed prior to defibrillation to secure good electrode contact. Arcing and burns may occur if electrodes or paddles are placed directly over a drug patch during defibrillation. After removing medication patches, wipe and dry skin before applying electrodes (Deakin *et al.* 2005).
- Ensure that there is no direct contact between defibrillation paddles and external pacing wires. Body jewellery, metal objects and medallions must be removed from the chest (Liddle *et al.* 2003).

Environmental considerations

- Petrochemicals or inflammable spirits or fumes can ignite with a spark so remove casualty to a safe area, if necessary.
- If the casualty is lying on a wet floor, covered in blood or vomit, he or she should be removed to a safe and dry area. The chest should be dried of any form of fluid that may conduct a shock.

Operator considerations

- The operator's hands must be kept dry.
- Paddles/gel pads should only be charged either when on the casualty's chest.
- Once defibrillation shocks are ended, the paddles must be replaced into their appropriate containers.
- The safety of bystanders and other staff is the responsibility of the person using the defibrillator. An audible verbal warning to all personnel to 'Stand clear' must be given by the operator.
- The operator must always perform a visual scan to ensure that nobody is directly or indirectly in contact with the casualty. Possible areas of indirect contact include any area of the bed-frame, infusion stands, electric cables and intravenous infusions.

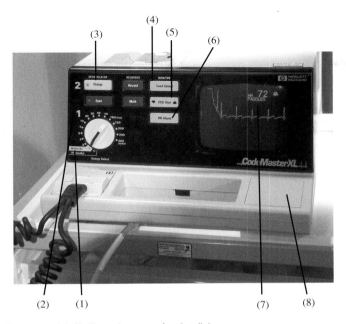

Figure 11.4 The manual defibrillator (see text for details).

MANUAL DEFIBRILLATORS

Manual defibrillators have been widely used but are now confined to critical care settings. They have some unique advantages over AEDs, including facilitating the operator to rapidly diagnose the underlying rhythm and to shock without waiting for rhythm analysis. This decreases the interruption of chest compressions (Resuscitation Council UK 2006). In addition, a typical device (as shown in Figure 11.4) has additional features that have the capacity to deliver synchronised shocks and provide external pacing. Most modern devices are also able to print a continuous rhythm strip and produce a record of the sequence of defibrillator shocks administered. All this activity can also be stored in a database. Defibrillator facilities may vary between manufacturers and therefore familiarity with equipment is mandatory; however, the main disadvantage of manual devices is that the operator needs to be skilled in cardiac rhythm interpretation.

(1) On/off dial;
(2) Dial to select energy required;
(3) Charge button – this may also be found on paddles;
(4) Button for selecting the monitoring of the ECG trace through leads only;
(5) Button to increase amplitude of ECG trace;
(6) Switch for setting upper/lower alarm limits;
(7) Cardiac monitor;
(8) Modern defibrillators also have a synchronise mode that is activated by a switch or button. This is selected *only* for cardioversion of atrial and ventricular tachycardias (see later in the chapter).

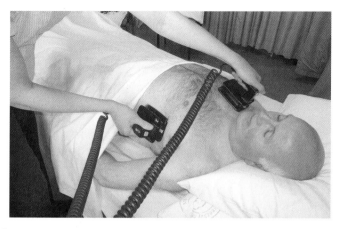

Figure 11.5 Operating a manual defibrillator.

Commonly, two other electrical cords leave the defibrillator and connect to an apex and a sternal paddle that are between 10 and 12 cm in diameter for the adult patient. When the power is on, pressing the paddles against the patient's chest will display the cardiac rhythm on the monitor screen (see Figures 11.4 and 11.5); in the cardiac arrest situation, this saves valuable time should the patient require defibrillation. If the patient does not require defibrillation, the ECG leads may then be attached.

Paddle design may vary, so knowledge of local equipment is vital. Figure 11.6 illustrates the usual functions available in handheld paddles.

(1) The sternal paddle is for selecting the energy levels (on some models).
(2) The apex paddle is the charge button and is activated when depressed (on some models); this must be while the paddles are on the patient's chest.
(3) To deliver a shock, both discharge buttons must be depressed simultaneously.

Familiarity with the equipment is important and testing of the device should be carried out daily. Box 11.2 provides a simplified procedure for performing manual defibrillation.

Limitations of manual defibrillators
(1) They are heavy and bulky.
(2) Operation requires additional training to achieve competence.
(3) Without practice, skill in operating a manual defibrillator and rhythm interpretation declines. Keeping updated requires time away from wards (Moule & Albarran 2002).
(4) Use has been confined to critical care settings, and only persons who have been certified as competent should operate manual defibrillators.

AUTOMATED EXTERNAL DEFIBRILLATORS
Modern AEDs have overcome many of the obstacles associated with manual defibrillators. Their ease of operation, technical reliability, use of voice and visual

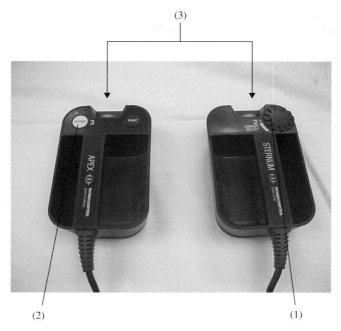

Figure 11.6 Defibrillator paddles (see text for details).

Box 11.2   Procedure for performing manual defibrillation.

The following sequence has been adapted from the Resuscitation Council UK (2006) guidelines in manual defibrillation.

- Confirm that patient has arrested, check breathing and pulse simultaneously.
- Confirm VF/VT from either the monitor or defibrillator paddles.
- Place defibrillator gel pads on patient's chest as recommended (see Figure 11.2).
- Select energy levels dial 150–200 J for biphasic or 360 J for monophasic defibrillators.
- Place defibrillator paddles firmly on gel pads (see Figure 11.1).
- Check that oxygen supply is at a safe distance of 1 m away prior to defibrillation.
- Keep handheld paddles firmly applied on the patient's chest and depress 'charge button'.
- Give a clear and loud verbal warning to 'stand clear'.
- Perform a visual scan to ensure that everyone is standing at safe distance from the patient.
- Deliver the prescribed energy shock.
- Keep the interval between defibrillation and chest compressions to a maximum of 10 seconds.
- If cardiac output is restored, replace paddles in their holders; however, should VF/VT persist, continue according to ALS algorithm (see Chapter 7).
- Monitor the cardiac rhythm through the ECG leads (Bradbury *et al.* 2000).

prompts mean that a broad range of first providers and rescuers can be instructed to safely attempt defibrillation in the cardiac arrest patient without delay. Since AEDs are programmed with dedicated software which can accurately assess the rhythm, the operator is not required to recognise or analyse cardiac arrhythmias (Resuscitation Council UK 2006). Due to these facilities, airline staff, paramedics and lay people with minimal training have been able to operate an AED successfully and safely (Capucci *et al.* 2002, Eames *et al.* 2003, Gottschalk *et al.* 2002, Page *et al.* 2000, Ross *et al.* 2001). Consequently, there have been recommendations that all healthcare staff should be trained to use an AED to reduce unnecessary delays to vital life-saving treatment.

SYNCHRONISED CARDIOVERSION

Defibrillators are also used to transform tachyarrhythmias of an atrial or ventricular origin into sinus rhythm, by selecting the synchronised cardioversion mode. Reasons for emergency cardioversion include:

- persistent atrial fibrillation/flutter;
- poor response or undesirable side effects from drug therapy;
- patient has become haemodynamically unstable due to a tachyarrhythmia;
- sustained supraventricular tachycardias which produce signs of cardiovascular distress (Trohman & Parillo 2000).

The aim of electrical cardioversion is to depolarise the myocardium, interrupt the tachyarrhythmia and so enable the sinoatrial node to regain control with a sinus rhythm. While the techniques and safety procedures for delivering the shock are similar in most respects, there are four major differences between defibrillation and cardioversion:

- use of anaesthesia;
- synchronisation mode;
- selection of energy levels;
- complications.

Use of anaesthesia

Synchronised cardioversion is usually a planned treatment and the patient's consent is required. Patients are starved for at least four hours and given a short-acting anaesthetic. Anaesthetic support must be present.

Synchronisation mode

For this procedure, ECG monitoring and all the essential equipment for managing CPR must be available. Prior to cardioversion the 'synch' button must be activated; this ensures that the shock is triggered to take place on the R wave and not with the T wave, as this will induce VF (Bennett 2002). If the complexes are small, increase the amplitude. Operators need to be aware of the delay between the time the discharge buttons were depressed and the actual shock; this is because the defibrillator is detecting a shockable R wave. Hence, the paddles must remain pressed firmly on the patient's chest and buttons depressed until the shock has been delivered. Some defibrillators default to unsynchronised mode after each shock. In others, the 'synch' button must be switched off.

Energy levels

- Monophasic waveforms – initial cardioversion energy levels for atrial fibrillation should start with 200 J, proceeding with incremental increases in energy levels.
- Biphasic waveforms – although rigorous evidence is unavailable, a reasonable strategy recommends that starting energy levels are between 120 and 150 J and escalating as required (Deakin & Nolan 2005).

Complications

- Systemic/cerebral embolism (with atrial fibrillation).
- Ventricular fibrillation.
- Transient rhythm disturbances.

Following the procedure, the patient must be placed in the recovery position until he or she regains consciousness. If the patient complains of residual chest pain, assess location, radiation, quality and intensity and administer prescribed analgesia accordingly.

IMPLANTABLE CARDIAC DEFIBRILLATORS

Implantable cardiac defibrillators (ICDs) provide superior survival outcomes when compared to traditional pharmacological interventions for specific patients who are at risk of sudden cardiac death from ventricular dysrhythmias (AVID Investigators 1997, Moss *et al*. 1996, 2002, Trappe *et al*. 1997).

ICDs are implanted subcutaneously via the transvenous route in the left or right deltopectoral area, similar to a permanent pacemaker. The procedure can be undertaken using local anaesthesia and intravenous sedation. An ICD comprises a generator (containing microprocessors, integrated circuits, memory boards and battery) plus one or more leads for pacing and defibrillation electrodes (Di Marco 2003, Tagney 2003). The software coordinates, senses, interprets, stores data and links with the different subsections of the system to provide an appropriate response (Pinski 2000). Current indications and guidelines for use are divided into primary and secondary prevention.

For primary prevention:

- non-sustained VT;
- inducible VT on electrophysiological testing;
- myocardial infarction, depressed left ventricular function with an ejection fraction (EF) of 30% or less (normal ejection fraction 65–70%);
- prolonged QRS equal or greater than 120 seconds;
- individuals at high risk of sudden death due to familial cardiac conditions: long QT syndrome or arrhythmogenic right ventricular dysplasia, Brugada syndrome.

For secondary prevention:

- survivors of cardiac arrest due to either VT or VF;
- spontaneous sustained VT associated with symptomatic haemodynamic compromise;

- sustained VT without causing syncope or a cardiac arrest in highly symptomatic patients who have an associated reduced EF (<35%) but whose heart failure is not totally debilitating (Houghton & Kaye 2003, National Institute of Clinical Excellence, NICE 2006).

Modern ICDs are highly sophisticated, with a battery that may last anything from five to nine years, and can be programmed to perform multiple tasks including:

- record intracardiac electrograms, allowing review of episodes of rhythm disturbances and defibrillation;
- arrhythmia detection;
- delivery of high-energy unsynchronised defibrillation shocks;
- discharge low-energy synchronised shocks (cardioversion) for VT;
- delivery of low- and high-energy shocks (tiered therapy);
- antitachycardia pacing;
- back-up pacing for bradyarrhythmias (Di Marco 2003, Pinski 2000).

It is important to know how to manage such individuals should the ICD fail and external defibrillation is required. Defibrillation can damage an ICD or pacemaker if electrodes are placed directly over the device. If defibrillation is required, it is advisable that:

- electrodes are placed at least 12–15 cm from ICD or pacemaker (Resuscitation Council UK 2006);
- use an anterior–posterior position for electrode placement;
- deactivate the device by placing a magnet over the ICD (Deakin & Nolan 2005, Pinski 2000).

Seek technical support to assess and evaluate ICD functions once the patient is stabilised.

REVIEW OF LEARNING
- ❏ Early defibrillation improves survival outcomes following a cardiac arrest; however, success is dependent on certain factors.
- ❏ Defibrillation is an emergency procedure that must be delivered promptly, effectively and safely.
- ❏ In the event of a cardiac arrest, if a defibrillator is not immediately available, CPR should be started at 30:2.
- ❏ The quality of CPR, in particular the depth of compression, prior to defibrillator-shock influences survival outcomes in VF
- ❏ Current practice recommends giving an initial defibrillation shock of 150–200 J (biphasic), or 360 J (monophasic) without reassessing the rhythm or pulse. If VF/VT persists, the advanced life support algorithm should be followed (see Chapter 7).
- ❏ Advantages of using an AED when compared to manual defibrillators include ease of use, rapid and safer defibrillation.
- ❏ Manual defibrillators allow for a more rapid assessment of cardiac rhythm and have other capabilities that AEDs do not have. A key disadvantage of manual defibrillators is that expertise in rhythm interpretation is necessary.

❏ Synchronised cardioversion is usually an elective procedure used to convert tachyarrhythmias of an atrial into sinus rhythm.
❏ Staff operating a defibrillator must always be aware of the potential dangers and hazards that may occur to the patient and bystanders while delivering a shock.

Case study

You are working a night shift and decide to get a snack from the vending machine. You arrive at your destination and hear a noise. Slumped on a chair, you find a gentleman whose shirt is soaked in coffee and who, when approached, is unresponsive to verbal commands or to gentle shaking of his shoulders.

What do you do next? Write down what you might do.

Make sure you and any bystanders are safe to approach. You check the victim for a response. If he does not respond then shout for help. Place the casualty on his back and open the airway with head tilt/chin lift. Look, listen and feel for breathing for up to 10 seconds. If he is not breathing, send someone for help or if alone, leave the victim and go to call for emergency help or ambulance. Deliver 30 compressions followed by two rescue breaths. Once the AED arrives, switch it on. While removing the patient's clothing, in order to place gel pads, you note that the casualty is wearing a long gold chain.

Write down what you would do next.

Remove all jewellery and, if wet, dry the chest as much as possible. Without interrupting chest compressions, place the sternal gel pad below the right clavicle and the apical gel pad should be positioned in the mid-axillary line, level with ECG electrode V_6 or female breast. Connect the cable to the AED.

What is your next action?

Follow voice and visual directions on the AED. The device instructs you to press the ANALYSE button but first make sure that nobody is touching the casualty. Within seconds, the AED confirms that the casualty is in a shockable rhythm. The voice prompt will then warn all personnel to stand clear. In the meantime, the AED will charge to a pre-set level; you may see this on the screen or hear an audible sound. You will then be advised to press the shock button(s). Before doing so, check your environment and make sure that everyone has stepped away from the casualty and that it is safe to press the defibrillation button. Once the patient has been shocked, the AED will reanalyse the rhythm. Proceed with CPR without checking for the presence of a pulse. If the patient remains in a shockable rhythm, follow the ALS algorithm (as in Chapter 7). Defibrillation was successful and the patient reverts to sinus rhythm with spontaneous circulation.

What should you do next?

Continued resuscitation after return of spontaneous circulation involves review of status using ABCDE system, further monitoring and investigations and safe transfer to an appropriate setting. During transfer, monitor the ECG, non-invasive blood pressure and oxygen saturation (see Chapter 14). Provide an accurate handover and document all relevant actions/interventions during the arrest and ensure the next of kin are notified.

CONCLUSION

Being a healthcare professional carries many responsibilities and the maintenance of competence in performing BLS and use of an AED can be regarded as one realistic expectation. Early defibrillation has been established as a major component of the Chain of Survival which, when administered promptly and safely, can have a positive and significant impact on patient outcomes. With newer devices being developed that are easy to use and safer, the scope for improving survival rates from cardiac arrest will increase. However, the challenge for all healthcare professionals is to keep updated and have the opportunity to practise regularly in order to be able to recognise and respond to a cardiac arrest call effectively.

REFERENCES

American Heart Association and International Liaison Committee on Resuscitation (2000) Adult basic life support. *Resuscitation* **46** (1–3), 29–71.

AVID Investigators (1997) A comparison of anti-arrhythmic therapy with implantable defibrillators in patients resuscitated from near fatal arrhythmias. *New England Journal of Medicine* **337**, 1576–83.

Bennett, D.H. (2002) *Cardiac Arrhythmias: Practical Notes on Interpretation and Treatment*, 6th edn. Arnold, London.

Bossaert, L., Handley, A., Marsden, A. *et al.* (1998) European Resuscitation Council guidelines for the use of automated external defibrillators by EMS providers and first providers. *Resuscitation* **37** (2), 91–4.

Bradbury, N., Hyde, D. & Nolan, J. (2000) Reliability of the ECG monitoring with gel/paddle combination after defibrillation. *Resuscitation* **44**, 203–6.

Capucci, A., Ascheri, D., Pieploi, M.F., Bardy, G., Iconomu, E. & Arverdi, M. (2002) Tripling survival from sudden cardiac arrest via early defibrillation without traditional education in cardiopulmonary resuscitation. *Circulation* **106**, 1065–70.

Chamberlain, D., Frenneaux, M., Stee, S. & Smith, A. (2008) Why do chest compressions aid delayed defibrillation. *Resuscitation* **77**, 10–15.

Coady, E. (1999) A strategy for nurse defibrillation in general wards. *Resuscitation* **42**, 183–6.

Cobb, L., Fahrenbruch, C., Walsh, T. *et al.* (1999) Influence of cardiopulmonary resuscitation prior to defibrillation in patients with out-of-hospital ventricular defibrillation. *JAMA* **281**, 1182–8.

Cobbe, S., Redmond, M., Watson, J., Hollingworth, J. & Carrington, D.J. (1991) 'Heartstart Scotland' – initial experience of a national scheme for out of hospital defibrillation. *British Medical Journal* **302**, 1517–20.

Cooper, M., More, J., Robb, A. & Ness, V. (1998) A guide to defibrillation. *Emergency Nurse* **6** (3), 16–21.

Deakin, C.D., McLaren, R.M., Petley, G.W., Clewlow, F. & Darymple-Hay, M.J. (1998) Effects of positive end-expiratory pressure on transthoracic impedance – implications for defibrillation. *Resuscitation* **37**, 9–12.

Deakin, C.D. & Nolan, J. (2005) European Resuscitation Council guidelines for resuscitation 2005 – Section 3. Electrical therapies: automated external defibrillators, defibrillation, cardioversion and pacing. *Resuscitation* **67** (suppl 1), S25–37.

Deakin, C.D., Nolan, J.P., Soar, J., Bottinger, B.W. & Smith, G. (2006) Advanced life support. In: Baskett, P. & Nolan, J. (eds) *A Pocket Book of the European Resuscitation Council Guidelines for Resuscitation 2005*. Elsevier, London.

Di Marco, J.P. (2003) Implantable cardioverter-defibrillators. *New England Journal of Medicine* **349** (19), 1836–47.

Eames, P., Larsen, P.D. & Galletly, D.C. (2003) Comparison of ease of use of three automated defibrillators by untrained people. *Resuscitation* **58**, 25–30.

Endelson, D.P., Abella, B., Kramer-Johansen, J. *et al.* (2006) Effects of compression depth and pre-shock pauses predict defibrillation failure during cardiac arrest. *Resuscitation* **71**, 137–45.

Faddy, S.C., Powell, J. & Craig, J. (2003) Biphasic and monophasic shocks for transthoracic defibrillation: a meta-analysis of randomised controlled trials. *Resuscitation* **58** (1), 9–16.

Gottschalk, A., Burmeister, M.A., Freitag, M., Cavus, E. & Standl, T. (2002) Influence of early defibrillation on the survival rate and quality of life after CPR in prehospital emergency medical service in a German metropolitan area. *Resuscitation* **53**, 15–20.

Gwinnutt, C., Coulumbo, M. & Harris, R. (2000) Outcome after cardiac arrest in adults in UK hospitals: effect of the 1997 guidelines. *Resuscitation* **47**, 125–35.

Harris, J. (2002) Biphasic defibrillation. *Emergency Nurse* **10** (7), 33–7.

Holmberg, M., Holmberg, S. & Herlitz, J. (2000) Incidence, duration and survival of ventricular fibrillation in out of hospital cardiac patients arrests in Sweden. *Resuscitation* **44** (1), 7–17.

Houghton, T. & Kaye, G.C. (2003) Implantable devices for treating tachyarrhythmias. *British Medical Journal* **327**, 333–6.

Liddle, R., Davies, C.S., Colquhoun, M. & Handley, A.J. (2003) ABC of resuscitation: the automated external defibrillator. *British Medical Journal* **327**, 1216–18.

Moss, A., Jackson, W., Cannom, D. *et al.* (1996) Improved survival with an implanted defibrillator in patients with coronary disease at high risk for ventricular arrhythmia. Multicentre automatic defibrillator trial. *New England Journal of Medicine* **335** (26), 1993–40.

Moss, A., Zareba, W., Hall, W.J. *et al.* (2002) Prophylactic implantation of a defibrillator in patients with myocardial infarction and reduced ejection fraction. *New England Journal of Medicine* **346**, 877–83.

Moule, P. & Albarran, J.W. (2002) Automated external defibrillation as part of BLS: implications for education and practice. *Resuscitation* **54**, 333–70.

Moule, P., Albarran, J.W., Bessant, E., Brownfield, C. & Pollock, J. (2008) A non-randomised comparison of e-learning and classroom delivery of basic life support with automated external defibrillator use: a pilot study. *International Journal of Nursing Practice* **14**, 425–32.

National Institute of Clinical Excellence (2006) *Implantable Cardioverter Defibrillators for Arrhythmias – Review of Technology Appraisal* 11. Available online at: www.nice.org.uk/nicemedia/pdf/TA095guidance.pdf (accessed 6 June 2008).

Pagan-Carlo, L.A., Spencer, K., Robertson, C., Dengler, A., Birkett, C. & Kerber, R.E. (1996) Thoracic defibrillation: importance of avoiding electrode placement directly on the breast. *Journal of the American College of Cardiology* **27**, 449–52.

Page, J., Kowal, R., Zagrodsky, J. *et al.* (2000) Use of automated external defibrillators by a US airline. *New England Journal of Medicine* **343** (17), 1210–16.

Pinski, S.L. (2000) Emergencies related to implantable cardioverter-defibrillators. *Critical Care Medicine* **28** (10, suppl), N174–180.

Resuscitation Council UK (2000) *Guidelines for the Use of Automated External Defibrillators: Resuscitation Guidelines*. Resuscitation Council UK, London.

Resuscitation Council UK (2006) *Advanced Life Support*, 5th edn. Resuscitation Council UK, London.

Ross, P., Nolan, J., Hill, E., Dawson, J., Whimser, F. & Skinner, D. (2001) The use of AEDs by police officers in the city of London. *Resuscitation* **50**, 141–6.

Soar, J. & Mckay, U. (1998) A revised role for the hospital cardiac arrest team? *Resuscitation* **38**, 145–9.

Spearpoint, K., McLean, C. & Zidemann, D. (2000) Early defibrillation and the chain of survival in 'in-hospital' adult cardiac arrest: minutes count. *Resuscitation* **44**, 165–9.

Tagney, J. (2003) Implantable cardioverter defibrillators: developing evidence-based care. *Nursing Standard* **17** (16), 33–6.

Tang, W., Weil, M.H. & Sun, S. (2000) Low-energy biphasic waveform defibrillation reduces the severity of post resuscitation myocardial dysfunction. *Critical Care Medicine* **28** (11, suppl), N222–4.

Trappe, H.-J., Wenzlaff, P., Pfitzner, P. & Fieguth, H.-G. (1997) Long-term follow-up of patients with implantable cardioverter defibrillators and mild, moderate or severe impairment of left ventricular impairment. *Heart* **78**, 243–9.

Trohman, R.G. & Parillo, J.E. (2000) Direct current cardioversion: indications, techniques and recent advances. *Critical Care Medicine* **28** (10, suppl), N170–73.

Valenzuela, T.D., Roe, D., Nichol, G., Clark, L., Spaite, D. & Hardman, R. (2000) Outcomes of rapid defibrillation by security officers after cardiac arrest in casinos. *New England Journal of Medicine* **343** (17), 1206–9.

Wanchun, T., Weil, M.H. & Shijie, S. (2000) Low-energy biphasic waveform defibrillation reduces the severity of postresuscitation myocardial dysfunction. *Critical Care Medicine* **28** (11, suppl), N222–4.

Whitfield, R., Newcombe, R. & Woollard, M. (2003) Reliability of the Cardiff Test of basic life support and automated external defibrillation version 3.1. *Resuscitation* **59** (3), 291–314.

Wik, L., Hansen, T., Fylling, F. *et al.* (2003) Delaying defibrillation to give basic cardiopulmonary resuscitation to patients with out-of-hospital ventricular defibrillation: a randomized trial. *JAMA* **289**, 1389–95.

Drugs and Delivery

John W. Albarran & Paul Snelling

12

INTRODUCTION

The most important interventions for successful resuscitation are the rapid initiation of effective chest compressions, ventilation breaths and early defibrillation. Currently, drugs have a secondary role and may be given to assist improvement of cerebral and myocardial functioning. Three of these, adrenaline, atropine and amiodarone, are currently included within the advanced life support (ALS) universal algorithm. Other drugs may be given for specific indications before, during and after cardiac arrest. However, there are very few drugs which are supported by a strong body of evidence (Deakin *et al.* 2006). The recent review of international resuscitation guidelines agreed to drop American names for certain drugs, e.g. *adrenaline* instead of epinephrine.

AIMS

This chapter reviews the drugs most commonly used during advanced resuscitation, including dosage and modes of delivery.

LEARNING OUTCOMES

At the end of the chapter, the reader will be able to:

❑ identify the *routes available for the administration of drugs* to support the circulation;
❑ describe the *mode of action* of the first-line drugs used in resuscitation;
❑ describe the *role of healthcare professionals* in administering drugs during a resuscitation attempt;
❑ state the *indications, contraindications and dosages* of other resuscitation drugs.

ROUTES OF ADMINISTRATION

During resuscitation, drugs may be administered to the adult by a number of routes:

- peripheral intravenous versus central venous;
- intraosseous route;
- tracheal route.

The intracardiac route for the administration of drugs is not recommended.

Peripheral versus central venous cannulation

Any patient with adverse signs of deterioration, who develops chest pain or becomes clinically unstable, should have intravenous (IV) access established. In the ideal circumstances, IV access should be achieved prior to the patient's condition worsening or suffering a cardiac arrest. The achievement of venous access is the most reliable method for administering drugs during resuscitation and therefore considered a vital component of ALS (see Chapter 7).

Peripheral cannulation is a skill that is currently performed by nurses and other healthcare professionals. However, inserting a peripheral cannula during a resuscitation attempt is not easy, because the patient's arms move with the motion of chest compressions and peripheral veins collapse because of reduced cardiac output. The usual advice to cannulate as peripherally as possible should be reversed; the largest available veins should be cannulated, most commonly in the antecubital fossa. If possible, a sample of blood should be withdrawn while cannulating and care should be taken with the disposal of sharps.

If the cannula is patent, drugs can be given through it at any time other than during defibrillation. All drugs should be flushed with 20 mL of normal saline and the relevant limb raised for 10–20 seconds to aid delivery of medication to the core circulation (Deakin et al. 2006). It takes up to 5 minutes for a drug, administered by a peripheral cannula to reach the central circulation during cardiopulmonary resuscitation (CPR). When compared to peripheral injections, peak concentrations and circulation times are shorter when drugs are given through a central route; however, insertion of a central venous catheter results in additional breaks in CPR and the risk of adverse complications. Hence, peripheral venous cannulation is favoured as it is quicker and safer and should not interfere with the performance of CPR (Deakin et al. 2006). In circumstances when a central line is already in situ, this should be the preferred route for drug administration during resuscitation. In other situations, securing central venous access should be performed only by experts and must result in minimal interruption of chest compressions (Resuscitation Council UK 2006).

Intraosseous route

If establishing intravenous access is difficult or is not possible, the intraosseous route should be considered. While this technique is commonly used in young children, it is also effective in adults. Drug administration using this route can reach similar therapeutic plasma levels within a timescale that is similar to an injection through a central venous catheter. Additionally, the intraosseous route enables the withdrawal of bone marrow, which can provide analysis of venous blood gases, electrolyte values and haemoglobin concentration (Deakin et al. 2006). In adults, the optimal routes for intraosseous access are the proximal and distal tibia.

Tracheal administration of drugs

If intravenous or intraosseous access cannot be achieved, certain drugs can be given by the tracheal route (see Table 12.1). However, due to concerns over unpredictable nature of drug delivery, concentration levels and identifying the effective dose for use during resuscitation, this option should be considered as a last resort.

Table 12.1 Drugs and tracheal route.

Drugs that can be administered via the trachea	Drugs that must not be administered into the trachea
Adrenaline	Calcium salts
Atropine	Sodium bicarbonate
Lidocaine	Amiodarone
Naloxone	

To achieve comparable therapeutic plasma concentrations to intravenous routes, the tracheal dose should be at least three times the IV dose. Prior to instilling drugs into the trachea (via a tracheal tube) these should be diluted with sterile water as this leads to better absorption (Resuscitation Council UK 2006). Pre-filled syringes are a convenient way of administering drugs via an endotracheal tube.

DRUG ADMINISTRATION

Recent changes in legislation now allow nurses and other non-medical staff to prescribe any licenced medicine including some controlled drugs, for any medical condition within their clinical competence (Department of Health (DH) 2006a, 2006b, 2007). However, patient group directives (PGDs) are still in place for use in certain situations and environments. Such developments aim to ensure that patients receive medicines in a timely and efficient manner, challenging the traditional hierarchy of healthcare provision. At present, only those who have successfully completed an independent prescribing course are permitted to prescribe any licenced medicine. Undertaking an advanced course in resuscitation does not authorise nurses or other non-medical healthcare professionals to administer drugs, during resuscitation, without prescription. Practitioners should be aware of and be guided by local policies for the administration of drugs and infusions. The fact that the patient has suffered cardiac arrest and there is a need for rapid response with the administration of key drugs should not excuse careful checking, and in being accountable for the actions and omissions. Nurses must be aware of the need to be guided by the Standards for Medicines Management (Nursing and Midwifery Council 2007).

Cardiac arrest trolleys must contain first-line drugs, ideally in the form of pre-filled syringes (see Chapter 4), for speed in preparation and ease of use. Vigilance when preparing and assembling pre-filled syringes (see below) is necessary. There have been calls for a standardised format for drugs kits (Jowett *et al.* 2001) but in the absence of this, staff should familiarise themselves with the contents of drug boxes on cardiac arrest trolleys. There are two types of syringes in common usage.

Pre-filled syringes

As the name implies, these are simply syringes which are pre-filled with the drug in its standard dose and diluted appropriately. To administer the drug, the box has to be opened, the cap is removed and then the drug is ready for injection (see Figure 12.1).

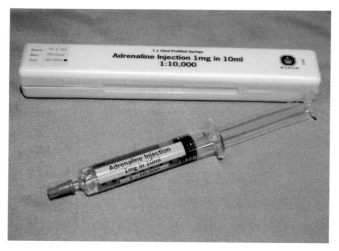

Figure 12.1 Aurum pre-filled syringe.

Min-I-Jet
These syringes (as shown in Figure 12.2a) require assembly immediately prior to drug administration. After emptying the components from the box, remove the protective caps (as seen in Figure 12.2b). The barrel and the plunger must then be screwed together (see Figure 12.2c). Finally, remove yellow hood, expel air and the syringe is ready for use (see Figure 12.2d).

Many of the drug dosages in the pre-filled syringes are standard, although this is not always the case. Practitioners should be aware that drugs come in different dosages.

DRUG CALCULATIONS
The dosages of resuscitation drugs are expressed in a number of ways and this can be confusing.

- Standard weight – for example atropine 3 mg.
- Solution strength – this requires both a volume and a solution strength to be prescribed; for example 50 mL of 8.4% sodium bicarbonate. Where a drug dose is expressed as a percentage, it means grams per 100 mL. So, for example, sodium bicarbonate 8.4% contains 8.4 g of sodium chloride in 100 mL of solution. Therefore, a 50-mL dose contains 4.2 g of sodium bicarbonate.
- Dilution – this also requires both a dilution and a volume, for example adrenaline 10 mL of 1:10 000. Where a drug is expressed as a dilution, it means grams in mL of solution. So, for example, adrenaline 1:10 000 contains 1 g in 10 000 mL; that is, 1 mg in 10 mL.

All drug administration during cardiac arrest must be fully documented to provide an accurate audit trail.

First-line drugs

Adrenaline

Adrenaline is a naturally occurring substance that stimulates the sympathetic nervous system (SNS). The alpha-adrenergic effect of adrenaline causes arteriolar vasoconstriction, redirecting blood flow away from the peripheries and thereby improving myocardial and cerebral perfusion pressures during cardiac arrest (Deakin *et al.* 2006). In addition, the rise in coronary blood flow influences the frequency of ventricular fibrillation waveforms enabling attempted defibrillation to promote the potential for the restoration of circulation. However, as yet there is no empirical evidence involving humans indicating that the routine

(a)

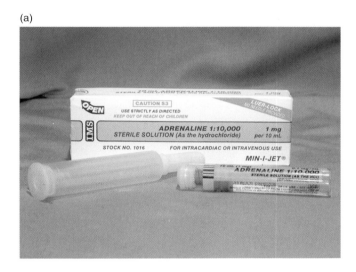

(b)

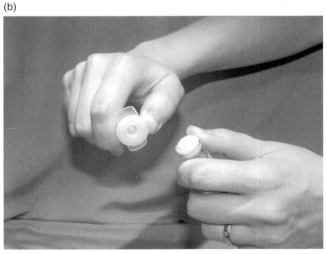

Figure 12.2   (a–d) Assembling a 'Mini-jet' injection for use.

(c)

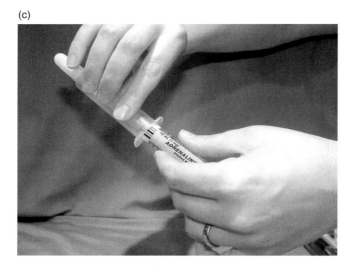

(d)

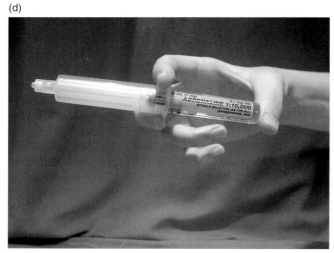

Figure 12.2 *(Continued)*

use of either adrenaline or any other vasopressor improves survival to hospital discharge.

Adrenaline is a powerful pro-arrhythmic and is very dangerous when given outside its limited indications (Johnstone *et al.* 2003). Due to difficulties in determining the ideal point at which to administer adrenaline, it is currently recommended giving this drug immediately after confirmation of the rhythm and prior to shock delivery (**drug-shock-CPR-rhythm check sequence**) (Resuscitation Council UK 2006). The principle behind this sequence is to allow adrenaline, which is given immediately prior to defibrillation shock, to be dispersed through the circulation by post-defibrillation CPR. During resuscitation, adrenaline injections should be prepared and ready to give to minimise interruptions to chest compressions and shock delivery.

Adrenaline for injection is supplied in two strengths: 1:1000 and 1:10 000. The concentrations are therefore 1 mg/mL and 1 mg/10 mL, respectively. Local protocols for the administration of adrenaline/epinephrine infusion should be consulted.

Dosages

- In a cardiac arrest, an initial dose of adrenaline 1 mg should be given if ventricular fibrillation (VF) or ventricular tachycardia (VT) persists following a second shock; thereafter, give adrenaline 1 mg every 3–5 minutes if the rhythm is unchanged (see Chapter 7). This is usually given by pre-filled syringe as 10 mL of 1:10 000 solution.
- In pulseless electrical activity or asystolic arrest, give adrenaline 1 mg once intravenous access has been established and every 3–5 minutes (or every other loop of the ALS algorithm, see Chapter 7).
- A low-dose adrenaline infusion can be titrated in the range 2–10 μg/min as an interim measure, while awaiting transvenous pacing for symptomatic bradycardia (see Chapter 10).
- In an adult or a child more than 12 years with severe anaphylaxis, an injection of 500 μg adrenaline (as 0.5 mL of 1:1000 solution) can be given intramuscularly. If there is no response, a further dose may be given at 5-minute intervals. Intravenous adrenaline can be given in extreme cases, but as this is dangerous it is only limited to **experienced specialists** (Resuscitation Council UK 2008; see Chapter 15). Electrocardiogram monitoring is mandatory.

Side effects

Unwanted effects include an increase in myocardial oxygen consumption and arrhythmias which may be further detrimental in the patient with cardiac ischaemia.

Amiodarone

Amiodarone is a complex drug, acting in many ways (Gonzalez *et al.* 1998). It works by increasing the duration of the action potential, though it also has anti-sympathetic and calcium channel-blocking properties (Taylor 2002). Amiodarone reduces membrane excitability and increases the refractory period; therefore, making cardiac cells less susceptible to transmitting ectopic impulses. Because of its unique pharmacological properties, amiodarone is effective in the management of both atrial and ventricular rhythms.

A number of studies have shown the effectiveness of amiodarone during cardiac arrest. In the amiodarone in out-of-hospital resuscitation of refractory sustained ventricular tachycardia (ARREST) trial (Kudenchuk *et al.* 1999), it proved better than placebo in terminating VF/VT. Similarly, the amiodarone versus lidocaine in pre-hospital ventricular fibrillation evaluation (ALIVE) (Dorian *et al.* 2002) reported improved results using amiodarone rather than lignocaine. Even if these trials did not demonstrate increased survival to discharge and beyond

(Taylor 2002), there is sufficient evidence to recommend the use of amiodarone in VF/VT cardiac arrest if the initial three-shock sequence has been unsuccessful.

Dosage

The dosages given will depend on the situation and administration should prefer-ably be via a central venous route. Current consensus recommendations include:

- If VF/VT persists after three defibrillator shocks, a 300-mg initial bolus of amiodarone diluted in 5% dextrose up to a volume of 20 mL should be given during rhythm analysis, then immediately followed up by a fourth shock of 150–200 J biphasic (360 J monophasic (Deakin *et al.* 2006). Pre-filled syringes are available for use.
- A further dose of 150 mg can be given for recurrent or refractory VF/VT to be followed by 900 mg infusion over 24 hours (Resuscitation Council UK 2006).
- Amiodarone is also effective in both broad and narrow complex tachycardias (see Chapter 10, Figure 10.9). If cardioversion has been unsuccessful and the patient's cardiovascular state remains compromised due to the underlying tachycardia, a loading dose of amiodarone of 300 mg should be given over 10–20 minutes followed by a further attempt at electrical cardioversion. The initial dose of amiodarone may be followed by 900 mg infusion over 24 hours.
- It should be remembered that all antiarrhythmic drugs are also pro-arrhythmic. Other specific side effects of amiodarone are corneal deposits affecting vision, hypotension and bradycardia.

Lidocaine

Lidocaine is indicated for refractory VF/VT when the first three-defibrillator shocks have failed to produce a return of spontaneous circulation and when amiodarone is unavailable (Resuscitation Council UK 2006). Lidocaine is a mem-brane stabilising anti-arrhythmic agent which acts by decreasing automaticity and of ectopic activity. It suppresses arrhythmias associated with depolarised cells (due to ischaemia or digoxin toxicity) with minimal disruption to normal tissue electrical conduction.

Dosage

- Lidocaine 100 mg (1–1.5 mg/kg) can be given as an alternative if amiodarone is not available; lidocaine should not be administered if amiodarone has already been given.
- A total dose of 3 mg/kg must not be exceeded.

Side effects are drowsiness, paraesthesia, confusion, muscular twitching and convulsions.

Atropine

Atropine is given to increase the heart rate and it works by blocking the ac-tion of acetylcholine at muscarinic receptors in the parasympathetic nervous sys-tem (PNS). Parasympathetic stimulation via the vagus nerve slows the heart. Blocking this in the sinoatrial (SA) node increases automaticity and there-fore heart rate. Blocking parasympathetic activity in the atrioventricular (AV) node facilitates conduction through the node and therefore heart rate. However, its value in asystolic cardiac arrest is inconclusive (Resuscitation Council UK 2006).

Dosage

The evidence base for the use of atropine in cardiac arrest is sparse; however, it is recommended for the following:

- For symptomatic bradycardia, a 500 µg of intravenous atropine should be given and repeated as necessary to a maximum dosage of 3 mg, the dose generally accepted to cause full parasympathetic blockade.
- Asystole and pulseless electrical activity (PEA) of a rate <60 beats/min, a 3-mg intravenous dose of atropine is recommended. This dose should be given only once (Deakin *et al.* 2006).

Side effects are dose-related and include dry mouth and blurred vision. In the elderly, confusional state may be aggravated after intravenous injection.

Magnesium sulphate

Low magnesium and low potassium levels can cause tachyarrhythmias. Intravenous magnesium sulphate is an effective and safe drug, which is useful for refractory VF/VT where low magnesium (due to potassium-losing diuretics) is suspected and in torsades de pointes (polymorphic VT; see Chapter 10). Other indications include digoxin toxicity and atrial fibrillation. The routine use of magnesium during cardiac arrest has not been shown to have a proven benefit.

Dosage

- For shock refractory VF, in the presence of hypomagnesia, an initial intravenous bolus dose of 2 mg (4 mL (8 mmol)) of 50% magnesium sulphate is recommended.
- In the case of ventricular tachyarrhythmias, in the presence of hypomagnesia, an intravenous dose of 2 mg of magnesium sulphate over 10 minutes is recommended.
- For polymorphic VT (e.g. torsades de pointes), an intravenous dose of 2 mg over 10 minutes is recommended (Resuscitation Council UK 2006).

OTHER DRUGS USED IN CARDIAC ARREST

Sodium bicarbonate

There has been considerable controversy over the use of sodium bicarbonate as a buffer to correct acidosis during cardiac arrest and there is little research to support its use (Bar-Joseph *et al.* 2002). Initial support for its routine use has diminished (Gazmuri 1999). Blood gas analysis is often unavailable quickly and in any case, arterial blood gases do not reflect intracellular values. In some cases, administration of sodium bicarbonate may worsen intracellular acidosis and reduce myocardial contractility (Adgey 1998). Additionally, some degree of acidosis increases cerebral blood flow, so normalisation of values may hinder cerebral protection. Currently, intravenous sodium bicarbonate (50 mmol, 50 mL of 8.4% solution) can be given in the following circumstances:

- cardiac arrest associated with hyperkalaemia (raised potassium levels);
- cardiac arrest associated with tricyclic antidepressant (for example dothiepin and imipramine) overdose;
- some experts advocate use of bicarbonate for severe acidosis – pH <7.1 or BE <10, but this remains controversial.

More accurate estimate of acid–base status can be determined by obtaining a venous sample of blood; if available, this should be obtained from a central venous catheter (Deakin *et al.* 2006).

Caution
- Sodium bicarbonate causes tissue damage if the cannula extravasates; a large vessel such as the external jugular vein is a preferred route for administration.
- A flush with 0.9% saline must follow sodium bicarbonate infusion.
- If given with calcium chloride, calcium carbonate is precipitated.
- The tracheal route must always be avoided as tissue may be damaged.

Calcium chloride
Calcium is vital for myocardial contraction. An initial dose of 10 mL of 10% calcium chloride can be given and repeated in PEA for:

- hyperkalaemia (high potassium levels);
- hypocalcaemia (low calcium levels);
- overdose of calcium channel-blocking drugs (diltiazem, verapamil and nifedipine);
- overdose of magnesium.

Side effects of intravenous calcium include severe tissue injury; if extravasation occurs around the cannula, reduce heart rate and stimulate rhythm disturbances. Avoid giving calcium, solutions and sodium bicarbonate at the same time and through the same venous access.

Adenosine
- Adenosine temporarily blocks conduction through the AV node. If a supraventricular tachycardia (usually narrow but wide if there is aberrance) involves re-entry within or through the AV node, adenosine can break the circuit, converting the arrhythmia to sinus rhythm. In the absence of a re-entry mechanism, adenosine stops the ventricles for a few seconds, allowing identification of an atrial arrhythmia. The period of ventricular standstill can be alarming for both staff and patient.
- When vagal manoeuvres have failed, a dose of 6 mg of adenosine, as a rapid intravenous bolus, should be given.
- If the rhythm persists, a 12-mg bolus dose can be given; if there is no resolution, a further 12 mg can be given. Rapid administration followed by a large flush is necessary.

- Cardiac monitoring is mandatory and facilities for recording the ECG should be available.
- Side effects are transient but unpleasant and include chest pain and hot flushes. Patients should be warned in advance.

Verapamil
- Verapamil is a calcium channel blocker, which can be effective in narrow-complex tachycardias (without evidence of atrial flutter).
- It should not be given where the origin of the tachycardia is in doubt (i.e. wide complexes) or in conjunction with beta-blockers.
- It can cause bradycardia and hypotension.
- The dose is 2.5–5 mg intravenously over 2 minutes.

REVIEW OF LEARNING
❑ The role of drugs during cardiac arrest is secondary to effective defibrillation, chest compressions and ventilation.
❑ Drugs have a supportive function in the management of cardiac arrest but there is limited scientific data to recommend their use.
❑ The preferred route for the administration of drugs during cardiac arrest is intravenously.
❑ Where IV access is impossible, alternatives should be considered, namely the intraosseous and tracheal routes. Appropriate adjustment of drug dosage is required.
❑ During cardiac arrest, IV adrenaline 1 mg may be given every 3–5 minutes.
❑ Intravenous atropine 3 mg can be given for asystole or PEA with a heart rate less than 60.
❑ A bolus dose of IV amiodarone 300 mg can be given for refractory VF and pulseless VT.
❑ Other drugs may be given according to the patient's condition.
❑ It is important to keep a record of all drugs and infusions administered during the cardiac arrest.

Case study

A 56-year-old patient admitted for clinical investigations for shortness of breath suffers VF, a cardiac arrest, and despite an initial defibrillation shock (150–200 J biphasic or 360 J monophasic) and CPR at rate of 30:2, the rhythm persists. After a two-minute cycle of CPR, another defibrillation shock (biphasic 150–360 J and monophasic 360 J) is delivered immediately after CPR resumes at a ratio of 30:2.

What drugs may be considered immediately afterwards?

Pause briefly after the last CPR cycle and check monitor; should the patient remain in VF, give 1 mg of intravenous adrenaline. This should be followed by a flush with sterile water. Once adrenaline has been administered, a third shock should be delivered (biphasic 150–360 J and monophasic 360 J: **drug-shock-CPR-rhythm check sequence**) and CPR should be resumed. After a two-minute cycle, the rhythm should be analysed for a brief moment and if appropriate, a further defibrillation. If VF persists following a third shock, a bolus dose of intravenous 300 mg of amiodarone. This should be given during a short pause for rhythm analysis with a 20-mL flush of 0.9% sodium chloride.

1.67 mL should be given (1.5 mL = 0.45 mg)

Make notes on the main function of the following drugs:
(1) adrenaline
(2) amiodarone
(3) atropine

What would you do? Record on the patient notes.
It is important to record the following information:

- time of cardiac arrest;
- number of shocks and energy levels used;
- drugs used, dosages and time given;
- initiation of any prescribed infusions currently in progress;
- whether any specific observations are required;
- contacting family members.

CONCLUSION

The evidence base for the use of drugs in resuscitation remains scarce and their role is regarded as secondary to the early initiation of CPR and attempted defibrillation. Nurses and other healthcare personnel, especially those in specialist areas, are increasingly able to recognise, prevent and manage cardiac arrests. Knowledge of the drug treatments available and sequence of use during resuscitation will enable responders to become more effective members of the cardiac arrest team; however, this should not compromise the ongoing maintenance and competence of key resuscitation skills.

REFERENCES

Adgey, A.A.J. (1998) Adrenaline/epinephrine dosage and buffers in cardiac arrest. *Heart* **80** (4), 412–14.

Bar-Joseph, G., Abramson, N.S., Jansen-McWilliams, L. *et al.* (2002) Brain resuscitation clinical trial III (BRCT III) Study Group: clinical use of sodium bicarbonate during cardiopulmonary resuscitation – is it used sensibly? *Resuscitation* **54**, 47–55.

Deakin, C.D., Nolan, J.P., Soar, J., Bottinger, B.W., & Smith, G. (2006) Advanced life support. In: Baskett, P. & Nolan, J. (eds) *A Pocket Book of the European Resuscitation Council Guidelines for Resuscitation 2005*. Elsevier, London.

Department of Health (2006a) *Improving Patients' Access to Medicines: A Guide to Implementing Nurse and Pharmacist Independent Prescribing within the NHS in England*. DH, London.

Department of Health (2006b) *Medicines Matters*. DH, London.

Department of Health (2007) *Safer Management of Controlled Drugs: A Guide to Good Practice in Secondary Care*. DH, London.

Dorian, P., Cass, D., Schartz Cooper, B., Gelaznikas, R. & Barr, A. (2002) Amiodarone as compared with lidocaine for shock resistant ventricular fibrillation. *New England Journal of Medicine* **346**, 884–90.

Gazmuri, R.J. (1999) Buffer treatment for cardiac resuscitation: putting the cart before the horse? *Critical Care Medicine* **27** (5), 875–6.

Gonzalez, E.R., Kannewurf, B.S. & Ornato, J.P. (1998) Intravenous amiodarone for ventricular arrhythmias: overview and clinical use. *Resuscitation* **39**, 33–42.

Johnstone, S.L., Unsworth, J. & Gompels, M.M. (2003) Adrenaline given outside the context of life threatening allergic reactions. *British Medical Journal* **326**, 589–90.

Jowett, N.I., Turner, A.M., Hawkings, D. & Denham, N. (2001) Emergency drug availability for the cardiac arrest team: a national audit. *Resuscitation* **4**, 179–81.

Kudenchuk, P.J., Cobb, L.A., Copass, M.K. *et al.* (1999) Amiodarone for resuscitation after out of hospital cardiac arrest due to ventricular fibrillation. *New England Journal of Medicine* **341**, 871–8.

Nursing and Midwifery Council (2007) *Standards for Medicines Management*. Nursing and Midwifery Council, London. Available online at: http://www.nmc-uk.org/aArticle.aspx?ArticleID=2995.

Resuscitation Council UK (2006) *Advanced Life Support*, 5th edn. Resuscitation Council UK, London.

Resuscitation Council UK (2008) *Emergency Treatment of Anaphylactic Reactions: Guidelines for Healthcare Providers*. Resuscitation Council UK, London. Available online at: http://www.resus.org.uk/pages/reaction.pdf.

Taylor, S.E. (2002) Amiodarone: an emergency medicine perspective. *Emergency Medicine* **14**, 422–9.

13 | Management of Potentially Reversible Causes of Cardiac Arrest

Rebecca Hoskins

INTRODUCTION

When a patient collapses suddenly and presents in cardiac arrest, it is vital to institute appropriate resuscitation measures. In addition, steps must be taken to identify the underlying cause, as this will enable the resuscitation team to implement strategies to reverse or correct the causative factors. The causes of cardiac arrest in the adult patient are attributable to airway obstruction, respiratory inadequacy and cardiac abnormalities (Resuscitation Council UK 2006), with many factors ultimately contributing to the subsequent cardiopulmonary arrest of the patient. Some, such as the obstruction of the patient's airway by the tongue falling back against the posterior pharyngeal wall, are easily remedied if the cause of the problem is identified quickly by accurate and timely assessment.

AIMS

This chapter explores the various causes for a cardiac arrest and describes the individual measures to reverse or correct the underlying problems.

LEARNING OUTCOMES

At the end of the chapter, the reader will be able to:

❑ list the *reversible causes* of cardiac arrest;
❑ describe how to *recognise and respond* to key causes of reversible cardiac arrest;
❑ demonstrate understanding of the *importance* of recognising and responding to the underlying cause of cardiac arrest;
❑ demonstrate understanding of the *non-reversible causes* of cardiac arrest;
❑ describe the factors that can influence a positive outcome in a cardiac arrest situation for the patient.

CAUSES OF CARDIAC ARREST

Cardiorespiratory arrest may occur because of a primary airway, breathing or circulation problem (Resuscitation Council UK 2006). However, it is important to remember that many life-threatening diseases can cause secondary respiratory or cardiac problems, which may ultimately result in the patient suffering a respiratory and/or cardiopulmonary arrest (see Box 13.1).

Box 13.1   Causes of airway obstruction.

Blood
Vomit
Foreign body, e.g. food or a broken tooth
Direct trauma to the face
Decreased level of consciousness
Epiglottitis
Swelling to the pharynx, e.g. caused by infection
Laryngospasm
Bronchospasm
Cardiomyopathy

Respiratory inadequacy may be due to disorders of the respiratory system such as asthma or pulmonary oedema. A decrease in the patient's respiratory drive may be due to central nervous system depression or decreased respiratory effort because of exhaustion or drugs depressing the patient's respiratory drive. In turn, the resulting hypoxia may have a direct effect on the heart by causing a bradycardia, which causes inadequate perfusion of the brain or heart and leads to cardiac arrest (Resuscitation Council UK 2006). Cardiac abnormalities may be a primary or contributory cause of the cardiac arrest (see Box 13.2).

A secondary cardiac abnormality is one where the heart is affected by a problem originating elsewhere (Resuscitation Council UK 2006). Thus cardiac arrest may occur following:

- asphyxia from airway obstruction or apnoea;
- tension pneumothorax;

Box 13.2   Causes of primary cardiac arrest.

Ischaemia
Myocardial infarction
Hypertensive heart disease
Valve disease
Drugs (e.g. antiarrhythmic drugs, tricyclic antidepressants, digoxin)
Acidosis
Abnormal electrolyte concentration
Hypothermia
Electrocution (which can cause paralysis of the respiratory muscles or send the patient into VF or asystole)
Cardiac failure
Cardiac tamponade
Cardiac rupture
Myocarditis

> **Box 13.3   Reversible causes of cardiac arrest, the four H's and four T's.**
>
> Hypoxia
> Hypovolaemia
> Hyperkalaemia/hypokalaemia (and other metabolic disorders)
> Hypothermia
> Tension pneumothorax
> Tamponade
> Thromboembolic
> Toxic/therapeutic disturbances

- hypovolaemia;
- hypothermia;
- severe septic shock.

The treatment of any potentially reversible cause of a cardiac arrest is of paramount importance irrespective of the underlying rhythm. The resuscitation guidelines (Resuscitation Council UK 2006) highlight the importance of considering reversible causes in *all* cardiac arrest rhythms.

The reversible causes of cardiac arrest can be most easily remembered as 'the four H's and the four T's', as shown in Box 13.3.

An important part of the process of resuscitation is the gathering of clues to piece together as much history as possible in order to elicit the cause or causes of the cardiac arrest. Thus, the team leader directing the resuscitation process may try to elicit further information about the events leading up to the point of cardiac arrest in the patient.

- Was there a history of trauma prior to the event?
- Does the patient suffer from any underlying disease processes, which may have been a contributory factor to their collapsed state?
- Does the patient take any prescribed (or non-prescribed) medication?
- Have environmental factors been a contributory factor to the collapse? Where was the patient found? When had they last been seen conscious by a witness?

MANAGING THE REVERSIBLE CAUSES OF CARDIAC ARREST

Hypoxia

Recognition
All patients who experience a cardiopulmonary arrest will have suffered some degree of hypoxia. Understanding the events leading up to the time of arrest will enable the team to discover whether it was the result of a primary cardiac event, such as a myocardial infarction, or whether it occurred at the end of a long period of physiological compensation. For example, the patient who experienced

respiratory failure as a result of a severe exacerbation of asthma will present with the following signs and symptoms.

- Tachypnoea (respiratory rate of greater than 30 breaths per minute or a respiratory rate of 10 breaths or less a minute).
- Exhaustion.
- Tachycardia or bradycardia.
- Hypotension.
- Reduced conscious level.
- Falling PaO_2, despite oxygen therapy.
- Rising $PaCO_2$, despite therapy (SIGN 2008)

Response

In order to prevent further hypoxia and to try to reverse the damaging effects of hypoxia on the myocardium, the patient needs to be oxygenated as effectively as possible. This may be achieved by ventilating the patient. This initially might involve a bag-valve-mask connected to high-flow oxygen (12–15 L/min) and ensuring adequate rise and fall of the chest.

- The gold standard is to secure the patient's airway with an endotracheal (ET) tube. However, expertise in this area is required and the hypoxia may be compounded while the ET tube is being passed. An alternative which may be considered in this situation is the insertion of a laryngeal mask airway (LMA).
- If the patient is intubated, it is essential that regular checks are carried out during the resuscitation to ensure the ET tube does not become misplaced into a bronchus or oesophagus.
- Misplacement of the ET tube will compound the hypoxia suffered by the patient.

Hypovolaemia

Recognition

The history precipitating the cardiac arrest may suggest severe volume loss, such as trauma due to rupture of the liver or spleen, gastrointestinal bleeding or rupture of an aortic aneurysm. The signs and symptoms of hypovolaemia are illustrated in Box 13.4.

Box 13.4   Signs and symptoms of hypovolaemia.

Tachycardia (rate >100 beats per minute)
Hypotension
Sweating
Pallor
Agitation
Thready or unpalpable distal pulses
Prolonged capillary refill time (>2 seconds)

Response

Replacement of intravascular volume is of paramount importance while advanced life support continues.

- For severe cases, a large-bore cannula should be placed into each antecubital fossa of the patient.
- The cannulae should be at least 16 G or 14 G in order to allow large amounts of fluid to be administered quickly.
- An alternative position for easy access is the external jugular vein of the patient. Two litres of crystalloid or colloid can then be administered as quickly as possible.
- There has been much controversy about the choice of fluid to be used in an emergency situation (Alderson *et al.* 2003). Saline 0.9%, Hartmann's solution or a colloid such as Gelofusin or Haemacel are all acceptable.
- The aim is to replace approximately 40% of the patient's circulating volume as quickly as possible.
- In high-dependency areas such as the emergency department, intensive care unit and theatres, infusion pumps may be available that can deliver 2 L of warmed fluid to the patient in less than five minutes.
- Having administered the fluid, it is important to remember to reassess the effect at appropriate intervals in the algorithm. This is especially important if the patient is in pulseless electrical activity (PEA), as a palpable pulse may then be felt after this intervention.
- If the underlying cause of the cardiac arrest was haemorrhage, urgent surgery may be required if the resuscitation is successful in order to stop the haemorrhage.

Hyperkalaemia, hypocalcaemia and metabolic disorders

Recognition

The cause of a cardiac arrest may be a metabolic disorder, often an electrolyte imbalance. The clinical history may alert the team to the underlying problem. Suspicion of the diagnosis may be confirmed through the measurement of arterial blood gases but serum electrolytes will provide more objective data (see Table 13.1). The ECG can also be used as an adjunct to the diagnosis.

- For example, if a patient suffered from renal failure, this may lead to suspicions of a raised potassium level. A 12-lead ECG taken previously may be helpful. Peaked T waves, broad QRS complexes and conduction defects are also indicative of a high potassium level (Soar *et al.* 2005), whereas ECG changes

Table 13.1 Normal serum electrolyte levels.

Electrolyte	Normal range
Potassium	3.5–5.0 mmol/L
Magnesium	>0.7 mmol/L
Calcium	0.85–1.4 mmol/L (with albumin corrected)

in hypokalaemia may include ST depression, flattening of the T wave and a prominent U wave (Soar *et al.* 2005).
- From the arterial blood sample, it is possible to determine the severity of acidosis following a cardiac arrest and also the measurement of key electrolytes, including potassium levels.
- If the patient presents having taken an overdose of calcium channel blockers, this may lead the team to think of hypocalcaemia being the cause of the cardiac arrest and this may be reversed by giving calcium chloride.
- In hypocalcaemia, signs and symptoms a patient may exhibit prior to cardiac arrest include convulsions, depressed cardiac function, muscle weakness, paraesthesia, tetany and ECG changes such as a prolonged QT interval (Womack 2002).

Response
- In all cases, continuous ECG monitoring should be instigated along with frequent observations and reassessment of the patient. A baseline blood test for urea and electrolyte measurement should be taken and this will be repeated at regular intervals.
- In hyperkalaemia, calcium chloride 10 mL of 10% should be administered intravenously in order to lower the extracellular potassium quickly and prevent any life-threatening arrhythmia.
- In hypokalaemia, potassium chloride can be given as prescribed, diluted in saline via a central line.
- In hypocalcaemia, 10 mL of 10% calcium chloride is given by slow bolus (Mahoney *et al.* 2005).

Magnesium abnormalities are frequently associated with other electrolyte abnormalities such as hypocalcaemia. Calcium and magnesium excretion are interdependent. Hypomagnesaemia can also cause refractory ventricular fibrillation and, if suspected, should be treated by giving intravenous magnesium to correct the electrolyte imbalance. Calcium chloride is also indicated if hypermagnesaemia is suspected (Womack 2002).

Hypothermia

Recognition
Hypothermia is defined as a core temperature less than 35°C (Soar *et al.* 2005).
   Mild to moderate hypothermia is defined as a core temperature of 30–32°C and severe hypothermia as a core temperature of below 30°C.

- If there is rapid cooling prior to the development of hypoxia, decreased oxygen consumption and metabolism may precede the cardiac arrest and reduce organ ischaemia (Gilbert *et al.* 2000). Therefore, becoming cold very quickly can exert a protective effect on the brain and other vital organs during cardiac arrest (Gilbert *et al.* 2000).
- Using a tympanic thermometer will give a fast reading to confirm the diagnosis. Oesophageal temperature monitoring may be used in a critical care area.

It is imperative to record the patient's temperature as soon as possible as it will directly affect the management of the cardiac arrest. If the first three shocks in pulseless ventricular tachycardia or ventricular fibrillation (VF/VT) are unsuccessful, then further attempts at defibrillation should be deferred until the core temperature is greater than 30°C (Resuscitation Council UK 2006), as they are very unlikely to be successful and will simply cause further damage to the myocardium.

In PEA, the ECG may show evidence of J waves. These are seen at the junction of the QRS complex and ST segments. They are thought to be due to hypothermia-induced ion fluxes causing delayed left ventricular depolarisation or early repolarisation (Nolan & Soar 2005).

Drugs should also be withheld until the core temperature is above 30°C, as administration will simply lead to pooling of the drugs in the peripheral circulation without any direct action on the heart.

Response

Once the diagnosis is established, passive rewarming methods such as using warm blankets will be ineffective if the patient has lost his or her cardiac output (Soar *et al.* 2005). Active and rapid rewarming is essential in order to reverse the cause of the cardiac arrest (Silfvast & Pettila 2003). Active rewarming includes:

- the administration of warmed (42–46°C) and humidified oxygen;
- administering warmed (40–43°C) intravenous fluids;
- catheterising the patient and carrying out a bladder washout with warmed fluids;
- peritoneal lavage with warmed fluid (which must be potassium free);
- the gold standard is extracorporeal blood warming (by-pass) but only a small percentage of hospitals can offer this treatment. It would be available only in centres where cardiac by-pass operations or haemodialysis are offered (Wollenek *et al.* 2002).

It is important to remember that during a prolonged arrest, a patient who was normothermic may become hypothermic (Resuscitation Council UK 2006).

Tension pneumothorax

Recognition

A tension pneumothorax develops when air enters the pleural space as a result of a laceration to the lung, bronchus or chest wall. The airflow is unidirectional, which means that air flows into the pleural space on inspiration but cannot escape during expiration due to the effective formation of a one-way valve. This causes a progressive accumulation of air in the pleura; the lung will collapse and the pressure will continue to build up, pushing the mediastinum to the opposite side. This in turn reduces venous return, resulting in a low or ineffective cardiac output (Greaves *et al.* 2001).

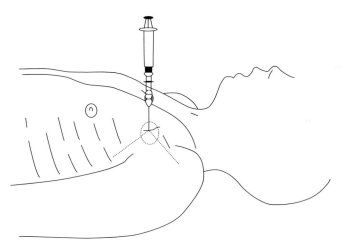

Figure 13.1 Landmarks for insertion of cannula.

Tension pnuemothorax is a clinical diagnosis. There is no time to confirm the presence of a tension pneumothorax through a chest X-ray. The signs which indicate a tension pneumothorax are:

- decreased or absent air entry in the affected side of the chest;
- hyper-resonance on percussion of the affected side of the chest;
- tracheal deviation (away from the affected side);
- distended neck veins (although this is absent in the hypovolaemic patient).

A tension pneumothorax may be suspected in a patient who has suffered chest trauma or asthma or has recently had a central line inserted.

Response
A needle thoracocentesis or needle decompression should be carried out by the medical team. A large-bore cannula is inserted into the second intercostal space in the midclavicular line on the affected side of the chest. Later on, a chest drain will need to be inserted (see Figure 13.1).

Cardiac tamponade

Recognition
In cardiac tamponade, blood fills the pericardial space which in turn raises intrapericardial pressure, compressing the heart and preventing it from expanding. As a result there is reduced cardiac output (Gao *et al.* 2004).

Clinical features of cardiac tamponade include:

- raised jugular venous pressure (JVP);
- hypotension;
- tachycardia;
- muffled heart sounds;
- pulsus paradoxus.

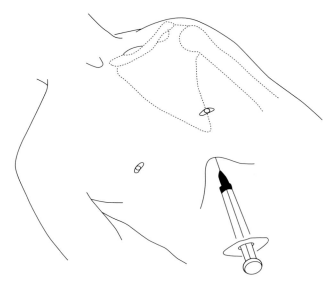

Figure 13.2 Pericardiocentesis.

The classic clinical features of distended neck veins, hypotension and muffled heart sounds are absent in cardiac arrest. The preceding history and an account of the mechanism of injury are therefore important. Suspicion should be aroused if the patient has suffered any trauma to the thorax and complains of chest pain.

Response
In order to treat this cause of cardiac arrest, a needle pericardiocentesis must be performed as an emergency procedure. An attempt is made to aspirate blood from the pericardial sac in order to enable the heart to fill again and produce a palpable cardiac output (see Figure 13.2). The patient would then need to undergo emergency cardiac surgery.

Thromboembolic or mechanical obstruction

Recognition
The most common cause of thromboembolic or mechanical obstruction causing the patient to lose his or her cardiac output is a massive pulmonary embolus. It has been suggested that an emergency pulmonary embolectomy (removal of the clot) can be life saving (Resuscitation Council UK 2006). In practice, this is not a procedure commonly carried out. There does appear to be a growing body of evidence that thrombolysis (giving clot-busting drugs) during the resuscitation may be helpful (Caldicott *et al*. 2002).

Signs of a pulmonary embolus before a patient loses cardiac output include:

- chest pain;
- shortness of breath;
- cyanosis;
- haemoptysis.

Table 13.2 Specific antidotes used to treat overdose.

Drug/poison	Specific antidote
Tricyclic antidepressants	Sodium bicarbonate if ECG changes occur
Opioids	Naloxone
Cocaine toxicity	Benzodiazepines
Beta-blockers	Glucagon
Organophosphates (weed killer)	Atropine
(Resuscitation Council (UK) 2006)	

Toxic/therapeutic disturbances

Recognition

Poisoning is a leading cause of cardiac arrest in younger adults (Resuscitation Council UK 2006). The drugs may have a negatively inotropic effect on the heart. Alternatively, cardiac arrest may be a secondary endpoint caused by respiratory failure or central nervous system depression (Soar *et al.* 2005).

There may be a definitive history of accidental or deliberate ingestion of therapeutic or toxic substances such as an overdose of tablets or exposure to carbon monoxide. However, even if there is no specific evidence of poisoning, it should be considered as the cause of cardiac arrest in every collapsed patient. The hospital team should ensure that they are not put at risk if chemical or radiation exposure from the patient is a possibility.

Response

- The emphasis is on intensive supportive therapy, with correction of hypoxia, acidosis and electrolyte disorders (Resuscitation Council UK 2006).
- If the ingested drug can be identified then the National Poison Centre can be consulted to see if a specific antidote is indicated (see Table 13.2). However, perhaps surprisingly, there are few specific antidotes available.
- An important factor to be taken into consideration is the fact that this group of patients is usually younger and therefore less likely to suffer from concurrent heart disease. The resuscitation may be prolonged as the poison may be metabolised or excreted during advanced life support (Resuscitation Council UK 2006).

Non-reversible causes of cardiac arrest

There are occasions when despite the best efforts of the resuscitation team, a positive outcome for the patient is not possible due to the primary cause of the cardiopulmonary arrest. Such causes may be divided into cardiac and non-cardiac pathology.

Cardiac causes

- Mitral valve prolapse.
- Hypertrophic myopathy.
- Massive myocardial infarction affecting a critical mass of myocardium.

- Continuous asystole despite advanced life support measures for more than 20 minutes in a normothermic patient.
- Patients who have received no resuscitation for at least 15 minutes after collapse.

Non-cardiac causes
- Massive trauma, such as massive cranial and cerebral destruction (Hillman 2003).
- Submersion in water for more than three hours in adults (Resuscitation Council UK 2006).

REVIEW OF LEARNING
- ❏ It is essential that effective basic life support and advanced life support are ongoing throughout a resuscitation.
- ❏ In order to aid a positive outcome, it is important to consider any or all of the potential reversible causes of cardiac arrest.
- ❏ These can be remembered as the 'four H's and four T's'.
- ❏ Even when every reversible cause is sought and treated, there may be occasions when despite the best efforts of the resuscitation team, the outcome for the patient is unsuccessful. This can particularly be the case when the cardiac arrest was caused by a catastrophic, irrecoverable event.

Case study

Mr Brown was admitted to the ward from the emergency department two hours ago. He has suffered from an exacerbation of asthma and was initially stabilised with continuous nebulised salbutamol. He was maintaining his oxygen saturations at 90–92% on 15 L of oxygen via a non-rebreathing mask. You go to administer a nebuliser and find him unresponsive and pulseless.

What are your actions?

On assessment of airway, breathing and circulation, the patient is found to be apnoeic and pulseless. The cardiac arrest team is called and basic life support is commenced. The monitor is connected and the rhythm is found to be PEA at a rate of 40.

What should be the actions of the team now?

The patient has been intubated and has received 1 mg adrenaline and 3 mg atropine. Cardiac compressions and ventilation are now being carried out continuously. (One potentially reversible cause of cardiac arrest has been addressed – hypoxia.)

Can you think of any other reversible causes of the cardiac arrest in this situation?

On reassessment, a thready pulse is felt. The patient is stabilised and moved to the intensive care unit for continuing care.

CONCLUSION

The seriously ill patient presents many challenges and being able to assess the signs of an impending cardiac arrest demands great skill. However, if preventive measures fail and the patient suffers a cardiac arrest, basic life support must be instituted as quickly as possible, followed by advanced life support. When it is established that the cause for collapse is not cardiac, but originating elsewhere, the additional underlying causes of the arrest must then be considered and addressed. Systematic analysis of the reversible causes of a cardiac arrest will enable rescuers to recognise the precipitating factors, intervene appropriately and influence survival outcomes.

REFERENCES

Alderson, P., Bunn, F., Li Wan Po, A., Li, L., Roberts, I., Schierhout, G. Human albumin solution for resuscitation and volume expansion in critically ill patients. In: *Cochrane Database of Systematic Reviews 2004*, Issue 4, CD001208.

Caldicott, D., Parasivam, S., Harding, J., Edwards, N. & Bochner, F. (2002) Tenectplase for massive pulmonary embolus. *Resuscitation 33*, 211–13.

Gao, J.M., Gao, Y.H. & Wel, G.B. (2004) Penetrating cardiac wounds: principles for surgical management. *World Journal of Surgery 28*, 1025–9.

Gilbert, M., Busund, R., Skagseth, A., Nilsen, P.A. & Solbo, JP. (2000) Resuscitation from accidental hypothermia of 13.7°C with circulatory arrest. *Lancet 355*, 375–6.

Greaves, I., Porter, K. & Ryan, J. (2001) *Trauma Care Manual.* Arnold, London.

Hillman, H. (2003) The physiology of sudden violent death. *Resuscitation 56*, 129–33.

Mahoney, B.A., Smith, W.A., Lo, D.S., Tsoi, K., Tonelli, M. & Clase, C.M. (2005) Emergency interventions for hyperkalaemia. *Cochrane Database Systematic Review*, CD003235.

Nolan, J.P. & Soar, J. (2005) Images in resuscitation: the ECG in hypothermia. *Resuscitation 64*, 133–4.

Resuscitation Council UK (2006) *Advanced Life Support Provider Manual*, 5th edn. Resuscitation Council UK, London.

Scottish Intercollegiate Guidelines Network & British Thoracic Society (2008) *Guidelines on the Management of Asthma.* Available online at: www.brit-thoracic org.uk/sign.

Silfvast, T. & Pettila, V. (2003) Outcome from serve accidental hypothermia in Southern Finland – a 10 year review. *Resuscitation 59*, 285–90.

Soar, J., Deakin, C., Nolan, J. *et al.* (2005) Cardiac arrest in special circumstances. *Resuscitation 6751*, S135–70.

Wollenek, G., Honarwar, N., Golej, J. & Marx, M. (2002) Cold water submersion and cardiac arrest in treatment of serve hypothermia with cardiopulmonary bypass. *Resuscitation 52*, 255–63.

Womack, K. (2002) Fluids and electrolytes. In: Newberry, L. (ed) *Sheehy's Emergency Nursing, Principles and Practice.* Mosby, St Louis.

14 | Post-Resuscitation Care

Ben King

INTRODUCTION

For every 100 inpatient cardiac arrests, approximately 45 will be successfully resuscitated and achieve return of spontaneous circulation (ROSC), but only around 17 are likely to survive to discharge from hospital (Gwinnutt *et al.* 2000).

The degree of existing acute and chronic disease and also the damage caused by the cardiac arrest will both influence short- and long-term survival; however, early recognition of problems coupled with a rapid response will increase the likelihood of a successful outcome (Langhelle *et al.* 2003). Post-resuscitation care should be thought of as continued resuscitation care and aims to stabilise cardiac performance, optimise tissue perfusion to the vital organs and minimise brain damage.

AIMS

This chapter describes the key principles of post-resuscitation care and approaches for improving long-term survival.

LEARNING OUTCOMES

At the end of the chapter, the reader will be able to:

❏ understand the importance of a *continued structured approach* to care of the patient in the post-resuscitation phase;
❏ demonstrate knowledge of the *principles of monitoring;*
❏ describe common methods of *monitoring the patient;*
❏ demonstrate awareness of *common post-resuscitation investigations;*
❏ describe priorities associated with *safe patient transfer;*
❏ discuss important issues relating to *care of relatives and staff* following resuscitation.

POST-RESUSCITATION TREATMENT

How unstable is the post-resuscitation patient?

The casualty sustaining a witnessed ventricular fibrillation (VF) arrest who receives a rapid shock to restore a normal rhythm may have had a cardiac arrest lasting less than 30 seconds and may not suffer any further complications. In contrast, some victims of cardiac arrest need lengthy advanced life support and require complex and aggressive management in the post-resuscitation phase. Factors affecting post-arrest physiology and outcome are detailed in Chapter 11 (see Box 11.1).

Post-resuscitation treatment aims to:

- optimise tissue perfusion, particularly of the heart and brain;
- identify the cause of cardiac arrest;
- prevent further cardiac arrest;
- enable safe transfer of patient to the most appropriate area.

Post-resuscitation management

Oxygen delivery to the tissues depends on proper management of airway, breathing and circulation. A structured assessment using the 'A–E' model (see Chapter 3) followed by a systematic approach to monitoring may allow recognition and response to any further complications in this extremely vulnerable group of patients.

MONITORING

There are some basic rules of monitoring, as seen in Table 14.1.

Airway/breathing

Observing the patient's level of consciousness, chest movement, respiratory rate and noise of breathing will all yield important information. This will be of even greater significance in association with recordings of, for example, blood pressure and heart rate.

Following a cardiac arrest, patients can be sufficiently alert to adequately maintain their own airway. Alternatively, some may have been intubated during resuscitation and will require the endotracheal tube to remain in place for a period during the post-resuscitation phase.

Table 14.1 Basic rules of monitoring.

Machines are fallible; always check the patient	• Poor contact of monitoring electrodes may cause a picture of asystole to appear on the monitor
Using machines to monitor patients does not replace basic clinical skills and close observation	• Changes in patient's mental status, skin colour and skin temperature will not be detected by cardiac monitoring and recording blood pressure
The readings and their significance must be understood by the nurse recording them	• Those caring for patients on cardiac monitors must have skills to recognise changes in rhythm and respond appropriately
Trends are more important than one-off measurement in determining whether patient is improving or deteriorating	• A heart rate of 60 beats per minute is likely to be entirely normal; however, it would be hugely significant if it had been 120 one hour earlier

Assisted ventilation may be required in the period after the cardiac arrest for the following reasons:

- apnoea;
- spontaneous breathing inadequate, breaths are too slow or shallow;
- oxygen and carbon dioxide levels require alteration and optimisation;
- patient unable to maintain required work of breathing;
- optimise the patient's cardiopulmonary status.

The process of respiration enables oxygen uptake and the removal of carbon dioxide. It is obviously essential to deliver adequate levels of oxygen in order to minimise tissue hypoxia, which can increase the risk of further cardiac arrest and also deprive the brain of vital oxygen supplies.

In certain circumstances, excessive assisted ventilation or hyperventilation by the patient can lead to a fall in carbon dioxide (CO_2) levels (hypocarbia). This can lead to a reduction in blood flow to the brain (Resuscitation Council UK 2000).

Oxygen saturation

Arterial oxygen saturation (SaO_2) describes the percentage of haemoglobin that is saturated with oxygen and is a useful measure of oxygen delivery. An SaO_2 of 97% indicates 97% of the total haemoglobin in the blood contains molecules of oxygen (Moore 2004). However, the patient with a low haemoglobin may have a very high oxygen saturation, even though the oxygen-carrying capacity of the blood is greatly reduced. Oxygen saturation monitors do not measure CO_2 levels nor do they offer any guidance on respiratory performance. The saturation sensor is usually placed on the tip of the finger or ear lobe. If perfusion to that extremity is reduced, the probe will not pick up a trace and will alarm for this reason and not because the saturation has necessarily dropped (Howell 2002). Other factors that can affect the trace include:

- patient movement, restlessness;
- dark skin pigmentation, jaundice and high serum bilirubin levels;
- blood, dirt or (blue or black) nail polish between sensor and finger;
- dysrhythmias;
- anaemia or abnormal haemoglobin.

Circulation

Inadequate circulation can be the cause or the consequence of cardiac arrest. It is essential to regularly assess blood pressure, pulse and respiration in order to recognise cardiac dysfunction and rhythm instability, which may follow a cardiac arrest and will require support until adequate perfusion has been re-established. It is worth noting that a rising respiratory rate is one of the earlier signs of circulatory failure.

Cardiac monitoring

As explained in Chapter 10 that the electrocardiogram (ECG) trace may be entirely normal in the presence of a cardiac arrest. This reinforces the point that the patient should be the focus of attention, not the monitor. Alterations in the rate

Table 14.2 Monitoring ECG changes.

Rhythm disturbance	Examples of possible cause
Irregular heart rhythm	• Hypoxia • Myocardial ischaemia • Heart block • Atrial fibrillation (AF) • Malfunctioning artificial pacemaker
Widening QRS complexes	• Rhythm originating in the ventricles • Bundle branch block • Electrolyte imbalance • Poisoning • Hypothermia
Lengthening PR interval P waves independent from QRS complexes	• Deterioration of AV node function • Absence of conduction across AV node (complete heart block)

and rhythm may be of cardiac origin or may reflect dysfunction in other systems, for example in the lungs or in electrolytes. Changes in the cardiac rhythm may be very dramatic and sudden, such as the onset of VF, or may be more subtle, such as a gradual rise in heart rate due to bleeding. The monitor will usefully detect changes, as seen in Table 14.2.

Central venous pressure monitoring

Central venous pressure (CVP) is the pressure in the central veins (caused by blood volume) as it enters the right atrium of the heart. It provides a measure of the circulating volume in the body. Measurement of the CVP assists the optimisation of pressures in the right and left sides of the heart. In right heart failure, fluids may be needed to stretch the right ventricle to make the heart work more efficiently. Alternatively, in left heart failure, diuretics and nitrates may be required to reduce the workload of the left ventricle, resulting in a predicted fall in CVP.

It is essential that all CVP measurements be taken from the same place, either the sternal angle or from the mid-axillae, where the fourth intercostal space and mid-axillary line intersect (Woodrow 2004). However, changes in patient position, hyperinflation of the lungs, overhydration and dehydration may also alter CVP readings.

Disability

The patient's neurological function should be assessed immediately after the return of spontaneous circulation. This should include:

- Glasgow Coma Score (see Chapter 16, Table 16.3);
- blood glucose.

Glasgow Coma Scale

Glasgow Coma Scale is used to assess and identify trends in neurological function based on specific body responses. Patients who are fully alert score 15 and those in a coma score 3.

Table 14.3 Commonly requested post-resuscitation blood tests.

Test	Reasons for test include
Urea and creatinine	• Assist assessment of renal function • Extent of dehydration
Blood chemistry	• Identify abnormalities in potassium, sodium, calcium etc.
Cardiac enzymes	• Identifying extent of cardiac muscle damage • Determining risk of ischaemic damage
Serum glucose	• Important to maintain at normal levels
Full blood count	• Identify risk or extent of bleeding

Exposure

Exposure and head-to-toe examination will be used to assess other aspects of the patient's existing pathology that may have caused or contributed to the cardiac arrest. Checking wounds, drains and the skin for signs of infection or dehydration may be of great significance.

Specialised monitoring

The following systems of monitoring are specialised and are most commonly seen in critical care areas such as intensive therapy units (ITUs).

Capnography

When a patient is intubated, a capnograph will measure the level of carbon dioxide in the exhaled air from the patient's lungs. Carbon dioxide is not produced by the stomach so the presence of CO_2 will assist in confirming that the ET tube is in the trachea and not in the oesophagus. Continuous capnography is not only a constant confirmation that the ET tube is in the correct place, for example during patient transfer, but will also reflect heart–lung function because if tissues are not effectively perfused only small amounts of CO_2 will be excreted. Thus, capnography reflects the adequacy of circulation (Schnell & Puntillo 2001).

Arterial pressure monitoring

This is a continuous and extremely accurate means of monitoring the systolic and diastolic blood pressure. It is used in critical care settings to assess the patient's response to the therapies given in the immediate post-resuscitation phase.

The pressures are displayed as continuous traces on a monitor.

INVESTIGATIONS

The same rules apply to investigations as to monitoring. There is no value to a 12-lead ECG or chest X-ray unless someone with experience is available to interpret them.

Twelve-lead ECG

ECG monitoring provides continuous information about the heart's electrical activity (see Chapter 10), whereas the benefit of a 12-lead ECG is that it produces 12 'views' of the heart and will record the electrical activity from three dimensions.

Additionally, not all heart-related problems can be displayed via a cardiac monitor so a 12-lead ECG is necessary to reveal these. For example, bundle branch blocks or myocardial ischaemia are easier to diagnose with a 12-lead ECG.

The 12-lead ECG can assist in investigating many clinical conditions, including:

- finer points of unstable rhythms and the conduction system;
- acute coronary syndromes (ACS);
- evidence of previous myocardial infarction (MI);
- structural heart damage;
- other conditions such as pulmonary embolus, chronic obstructive pulmonary disease, digoxin toxicity, electrolyte disorders.

Blood tests

A great many tests may be conducted on blood taken from the post-arrest patient (see Table 14.3).

Arterial blood gases

All the tests listed in Table 14.3 are usually measured from a blood sample from a vein (venous). By definition, an arterial blood sample is taken from an artery. Blood pressure in the arteries is much higher than in the veins so bleeding occurs from the puncture site more profusely and for much longer and so firm pressure for an extended time is required after the sample is taken.

The arterial blood gas (ABG) is used to:

- evaluate derangements of acid–base balance;
- establish levels of blood oxygenation and CO_2 elimination;
- assess whether the underlying problem is respiratory or metabolic.

Normal metabolism creates a slight excess of acidic compounds, which are normally excreted by the kidneys and also the process of respiration. Cells of the body require a degree of acidosis/alkalosis that is normal or close to normal (Driscoll *et al.* 1997).

During a cardiac arrest, an acidaemia is likely to develop due to:

- build-up of lactic acid as the tissues are starved of oxygen (metabolic);
- build-up of CO_2 as it cannot be removed by the lungs (respiratory).

The post-arrest patient is highly likely to be suffering from an acidaemia that is both metabolic and respiratory in origin.

Chest X-ray

In this situation, the chest X-ray is used to look for pathology that may have caused the cardiac arrest or any potential damage resulting from the resuscitation (see Table 14.4).

TRANSFER

It is almost certain that the patient who has sustained a cardiac arrest will need to be transferred following the event. Even if the cardiac arrest occurred in an environment, such as the intensive care unit (ICU), the patient may require transfer

Table 14.4 Chest X-ray assessment.

Lungs	• Pneumothorax or haemothorax
	• Pulmonary oedema
	• Pleural effusion
Heart	• Size and shape will assist diagnosis of heart failure
Bones	• Rib fractures
Tubes and lines inserted during resuscitation	• ET tube
	• Central venous line
	• Nasogastric tube
	• Temporary pacing wire

to theatre and/or X-ray for diagnostic imaging. Regardless method of transport, it is difficult to estimate how long patient transfer may last and staff should be equipped to deal with every situation.

Stabilisation prior to departure

Prior to departure, the team leader must ensure that the patient's airway, breathing and circulation have been stabilised. Experienced personnel must be available to ensure that the patient transfer is well co-ordinated and managed.

Patient transfer is a dangerous time for a number of reasons:

- less support available from experienced colleagues;
- poor working environment, space and light;
- movement may displace tubes and lines;
- often less equipment, only limited amount can be carried;
- if something breaks or oxygen runs out, difficult to replace;
- it may not have been possible to completely stabilise airway, breathing and circulation.

Equipment and staff

Due to the possible dangers associated with patient transfer, potential complications will have to be considered and plans drawn up. All necessary equipment to monitor the patient and effectively manage airway, breathing and circulation must accompany the patient along with appropriately skilled staff. The Intensive Care Society has set national standards for the transfer of the critically ill adult (Intensive Care Society 2002).

Communication and documentation

Communication between the transfer team and the receiving unit/department is paramount. Those receiving the patient need to be informed as to why and when the transfer is happening. The information required prior to transfer should include personal details of the patient, past medical history and reason for transfer. The nature of the patient's clinical condition must also be communicated so that staff at the receiving end can prepare the bed space accordingly.

It is generally good practice to have clear written summaries of events that have taken place, but in the case of a patient transfer, it is essential. All relevant notes, scans, results and charts should be made available to the receiving unit

Table 14.5 Levels of classification.

Level 0	Needs can be met by normal ward care within an acute hospital
Level 1	Needs can be met on acute ward with advice and support from critical care team
Level 2	Requiring detailed observation or intervention due to single failing organ system
Level 3	Requiring advanced ventilatory support together with support of more than one organ system

along with clear summaries of what has taken place. Cardiac arrest audit forms should be completed after resuscitation events, to allow analysis of where/when cardiac arrests are happening, their management and outcome. These are usually returned to the hospital resuscitation officer.

Definitive placement: where should the patient be managed?
The level of life support required will determine the placement of the patient after a cardiac arrest. A classification of critical care patients was published by the Department of Health (DH 2000) as part of a review of critical care services (see Table 14.5).

Rarely will post-arrest patients be anything other than level 2 or 3 unless they either have a 'do not attempt resuscitation' (DNAR) order made or have active treatment withdrawn. Patients who have cardiac disease will usually be cared for in a coronary care unit (CCU) even if they require complex management. As stated in the classification, ITUs are for those who need ventilation and/or have multi-system failure.

PREDICTION OF OUTCOME
Return of spontaneous circulation is obviously a favourable outcome from cardiac arrest but significant numbers of these patients do not survive to hospital discharge. It would be advantageous, for both the patient and their relatives, if it were possible to predict in the immediate post-resuscitation phases whether or not long-term survival was likely or even possible.

It would be unethical to deny patients ongoing care if survival was possible so any method that predicts outcome must be entirely reliable. No tests currently exist to determine outcome in the first few hours (Resuscitation Council UK and ERC 2000). Various types of tests and investigations are under review, including blood tests (levels of S-100 protein) and assessment of activity in the brain (electroencephalograph, EEG). Assessment at three days is of far greater reliability than immediately after circulation is restored.

Therapeutic hypothermia
Recently published research has confirmed that mild hypothermia in the 24 hours following an out-of-hospital VF arrest is beneficial to neurological function (Bernard *et al.* 2002). The study subjects who were cooled to 34°C had a significantly better neurological performance than those in the control group who were not cooled. This has led the International Liaison Committee on Resuscitation to issue a statement that unconscious adult survivors of out-of-hospital VF arrest should be cooled to 32–34°C for 12–24 hours (Nolan *et al.* 2003). The statement

also suggests that cooling may assist neurological recovery from cardiac arrests in hospital or from those with other presenting rhythms.

Post-resuscitation therapeutic cooling has become standard therapy in many ICUs and devices have been developed to help achieve this.

CARE OF PATIENT'S RELATIVES

Breaking bad news
The issue of breaking bad news to relatives is extremely important and should be undertaken by a senior and experienced member of staff. Conversations of this nature should take place in a quiet room without interruption. Relatives must be allowed time to reflect on the news and to ask any questions they wish. The news may be devastating even if the cardiac arrest had occurred after a lengthy and serious period of illness. Several sensitive issues may need to be broached with the relatives, such as whether or not a postmortem is required and the possibility of organ donation (Department for Work and Pensions 2003).

Postmortem
If the cause of death cannot be established or the doctors wish to know more about the cause of death, the coroner may require that funeral arrangements are delayed until a postmortem has been performed. The consent of relatives is not needed but they are entitled to be represented at the examination by a doctor.

Organ donation
If the resuscitation has failed but there is a possibility that the patient's organs or tissue are suitable for donation, the transplant team needs to be involved. Likewise, if the deceased patient had expressed a wish for their organs to be donated, the transplant co-ordinator should be contacted as soon as possible. Should a family member be present, he or she will be consulted about taking this forward.

The following organs are usually taken from donors who have been certified brain dead but who are ventilated in an ICU.

- Kidneys
- Heart
- Lungs
- Liver
- Pancreas

The following can be removed up to the following times after death.

- Corneas – up to 24 hours
- Skin – up to 24 hours
- Bone – up to 36 hours
- Heart valves – up to 72 hours

Spiritual needs/last offices
Those relatives with specific religious or spiritual beliefs may request contact with a priest or representative of a particular faith. The hospital chaplaincy can help

to organise contact. These contacts are not only comforting for relatives but are useful and sometimes necessary as certain faiths have strict requirements as to what happens to the body immediately after death.

CARE OF THE STAFF

Cardiac arrests, particularly on wards where they happen infrequently, can have implications for staff. It is essential that those involved with these extremely stressful situations are given the opportunity for discussion afterwards. They may find it useful to talk through the event and to have questions and concerns addressed. There are often feelings of guilt ('I should have got help sooner') or anger ('Why wasn't the patient allowed to die with dignity?'). These feelings may subside if an honest discussion takes place. For very unexpected and traumatic situations, counselling services or even clinical psychologists may assist staff in coming to terms with these events.

REVIEW OF LEARNING

❏ A structured assessment using the 'A–E' model followed by monitoring supports the recognition of and response to any further cardiac arrests.
❏ Common monitoring includes capnography and arterial pressure monitoring.
❏ Investigations will often include 12-lead ECG, blood tests, arterial blood gases and chest X-ray.
❏ Casualties should be stabilised prior to transfer.
❏ Relatives and staff will require support in the post-resuscitation phase.

Case study

In the week following major surgery, the patient develops signs of dehydration and evidence of worsening infection. The patient subsequently suffers a pulseless electrical activity (PEA) cardiac arrest. The post-arrest team must take into account the management of both potential hypovolaemia and sepsis.

Using the A–E model, discuss what you would monitor in such a patient.

- Airway – look, listen and feel for signs of airway obstruction, ensure airway remains patent potentially using positioning, suction and simple devices.
- Breathing – gauge whether breathing is effective, checking rate and depth, monitor signs of decreased respiratory effort and effects of inadequate oxygenation such as changing heart rate, falling oxygen saturation.
- Circulation – assess signs of adequate circulation by monitoring heart rate, pulse volume, blood pressure, capillary refill and peripheral temperature.
- Disability – monitor level of consciousness using the Glasgow Coma Scale or AVPU scoring system.
- Exposure – look at the patient, checking urine output, wounds and drainage. Look for signs of bleeding and infection.

As a team member, discuss which aspects you would consider in planning the care and management of the patient.

To conclusively confirm hypovolaemia, a CVP will be placed. Management of hypovolaemia requires fluid replacement (blood, plasma or crystalloids) while avoiding fluid overload. Sepsis may exacerbate hypovolaemia by vasodilation and capillary leakage.

It is important to remember that this patient's history does not exclude the possibility of a cardiac arrest secondary to an MI. The patient is likely to require a period of time on a ventilator in the ITU. This will allow assessment and optimisation of heart function, effective management of any infection and support to other systems such as renal function whilst ensuring adequate hydration and nutrition.

CONCLUSION

A significant proportion of cardiac arrest casualties do regain a spontaneous circulation but do not survive to discharge from hospital. This group requires effective continuing care in the post-resuscitation phase to maximise survival chances. Complex management may be necessary alongside careful observation and a series of investigations before the patient is stabilised. If patient transfer is required, only those with experience and expertise must be involved. It is also important to remember that, following a resuscitation event, both the patient's relatives and members of staff may need emotional support.

REFERENCES

Bernard, S., Gray, T., Buist, M. *et al.*, for the HACA Study Group (2002) Mild therapeutic hypothermia to improve the neurologic outcome after cardiac arrest. *New England Journal of Medicine* **346**, 549–54.

Department of Health (2000) *Comprehensive Critical Care – A Review of Adult Critical Care Services.* Department of Health, London.

Department for Work and Pensions (2003) *What to Do After a Death in England and Wales – A Guide to What You Must Do and the Help You Can Get.* Department for Work and Pensions, London.

Driscoll, P., Brown, T., Gwinnutt, C. & Wardle, T. (1997) *A Simple Guide to Blood Gas Analysis.* BMJ Books, London.

Gwinnutt, C., Columb, M. & Harris, R. (2000) Outcome after cardiac arrest in hospitals: effect of 1997 guidelines. *Resuscitation* **47**, 125–35.

Howell, M. (2002) The correct use of pulse oximetry in measuring oxygen status. *Professional Nurse* **17** (7), 416–18.

Intensive Care Society (2002) *Guidelines for the Transfer of the Critically Ill Adult*, 2nd edn. Available online at: www.ics.ac.uk/downloads/icstransport2002mem.pdf.

Langhelle, A., Tyvold, S.S., Lexow, K., Hapnes, S.A., Sunde, K. & Steen, P.A. (2003) In-hospital factors associated with improved outcome after out-of-hospital cardiac arrest. A comparison between four regions in Norway. *Resuscitation* **56**, 247–63.

Moore, T. (2004) Pulse oximetry. In: Moore, T. & Woodrow, P. (eds) *High Dependency Nursing Care.* Routledge, London.

Nolan, J.P., Morley, P.T., Vanden Hoek, T.L., Hickey, R.W., for the ALS Task Force (2003) Therapeutic hypothermia after cardiac arrest. An advisory statement by the Advanced Life Support Task Force of the International Liaison Committee on Resuscitation. *Resuscitation* **57**, 231–5.

Resuscitation Council UK (2000) *Advanced Life Support Course Provider Manual*, 4th edn. Resuscitation Council UK, London.

Schnell, H. & Puntillo, K. (2001) *Critical Care Nursing Secrets.* Hanley & Belfus Inc, Philadelphia.

Woodrow, P. (2004) Central venous pressure and cardiac output studies. In: Moore, T. & Woodrow, P. (eds) *High Dependency Nursing Care.* Routledge, London.

Special Circumstances

15

Jackie Younker

INTRODUCTION

The advanced life support algorithm provides a sequence of actions for the management of cardiac arrest. However, there are circumstances in which the team may need to modify its approach to meet the needs of the individual victim. Recognising pre-monitory signs and responding with prompt treatment may prevent cardiac arrest in these situations. A large proportion of cardiac arrests in younger people who do not have coexisting cardiac disease are due to special circumstances. It is essential to provide early and effective resuscitation to offer the best chance of survival. The circumstances covered in this chapter are:

- anaphylaxis;
- asthma;
- drowning;
- electrocution;
- hypothermia;
- poisoning and drug overdose;
- pregnancy.

AIMS

This chapter discusses how cardiopulmonary resuscitation (CPR) attempts should be modified in special circumstances.

LEARNING OUTCOMES

At the end of the chapter, the reader will be able to:

- ❏ recognise special circumstances that may require *modification in resuscitation techniques*;
- ❏ respond to *special emergency situations* appropriately and effectively;
- ❏ discuss *modifications in basic and advanced life support* to meet the needs of the individual casualty and their specific circumstances.

ANAPHYLAXIS

The annual incidence of anaphylaxis is increasing and probably associated with a significant rise in the prevalence of allergic disease over the last two or three decades. Anaphylaxis is a severe, life-threatening, generalised or systemic

Table 15.1 Possible causes of anaphylaxis.

Insect stings, drugs, contrast media, some foods (milk, eggs, fish and shellfish)	Most common causes of anaphylaxis
Peanut and nut allergies	Recognised as particularly dangerous
Aspirin, non-steroidal anti-inflammatory agents, parenteral penicillins and vaccines	Notorious causes of anaphylaxis
Beta-blockers	May increase the incidence and severity of anaphylaxis and antagonise the response to epinephrine

hypersensitivity reaction. This reaction is usually unexpected and is characterised by rapidly developing life-threatening airway and/or breathing and/or circulation problems usually associated with skin and mucosal changes (Resuscitation Council UK 2008). Table 15.1 offers a list of possible causes of anaphylaxis.

Recognising anaphylaxis

Anaphylaxis is not always recognised. The lack of any consistent clinical manifestation and a range of possible presentations make it difficult to diagnose. Inappropriate adrenaline injections are given to patients for simple allergic reactions that just involved the skin, or vasovagal reactions or panic attacks. Guidance based on the emergency treatment of anaphylactic reactions (Resuscitation Council UK 2008) suggests the following key points to help with recognition and prompt appropriate treatment.

- Anaphylaxis is likely if a patient who is exposed to a trigger (refer to Table 15.1) develops a sudden illness (usually within minutes of exposure) with rapidly progressing skin changes and life-threatening airway and/or breathing and/or circulation problems.

*Anaphylaxis is likely when **all** of the following three criteria are met*:

- sudden onset and rapid progression of symptoms;
- life-threatening airway and/or breathing and/or circulation problems;
- skin and/or mucosal changes (flushing, urticaria and angioedema).

Exposure to a known allergen for the patient supports the diagnosis. Skin and mucosal changes alone are not a sign of an anaphylactic reaction. Skin and mucosal changes can be subtle or absent in up to 20% or reactions (some patients may only have a circulation problem such as low blood pressure). There may also be gastrointestinal symptoms (vomiting, abdominal pain and incontinence).

Look for a sudden onset and rapid progression of symptoms:

- the patient will look and feel unwell;
- reactions occur over several minutes in most cases;
- intravenous (IV) triggers will cause a faster onset reaction than stings which, in turn, tend to cause a faster onset than triggers that are ingested orally;
- patients usually feel anxious and a 'sense of impending doom'.

The ABCDE approach to patient assessment is described in Chapter 3 and should be used to recognise life-threatening airway, breathing and circulation problems.

Airway problems:

- airway swelling (e.g. throat and tongue swelling). The patient may complain of difficulty in breathing and swallowing with a feeling the throat is closing up;
- hoarse voice;
- stridor – a high-pitched noise heard during inspiration caused by upper airway obstruction.

Breathing problems:

- increased respiratory rate;
- shortness of breath;
- wheeze – a 'whistling' noise heard during inspiration or expiration caused by airway narrowing;
- patient becoming tired;
- confusion caused by hypoxia;
- cyanosis – this is usually a late sign;
- respiratory arrest.

Circulation problems:

- signs of shock – pale, clammy;
- feeling faint (dizziness), collapse;
- increased pulse rate;
- low blood pressure;
- decreased conscious level or loss of consciousness;
- myocardial ischaemia and electrocardiograph (ECG) changes may occur even in individuals with normal coronary arteries;
- cardiac arrest.

The airway, breathing and circulation problems may cause decreased brain perfusion and alter the patient's neurologic status (*Disability problems*). Signs include confusion, agitation and loss of consciousness.

Skin and mucosal changes should be assessed as part of the *Exposure* when using the ABCDE approach.

- Skin changes present in over 80% of anaphylactic reactions and are often the first feature.
- They can be subtle or dramatic.
- There may be just skin, just mucosal, or both skin and mucosal changes.
- Erythema – a patchy or generalised red rash may be present.
- Urticaria – also called hives, nettle rash, weals or welts can appear anywhere on the body.
- Angioedema – similar to urticaria but involves swelling of deeper tissues, most commonly in the eyelids and lips, and sometimes in the mouth and throat.

Responding to anaphylaxis

The diagnosis of anaphylaxis is not always obvious. All those who treat patients having an anaphylactic reaction must use the systematic ABCDE approach and

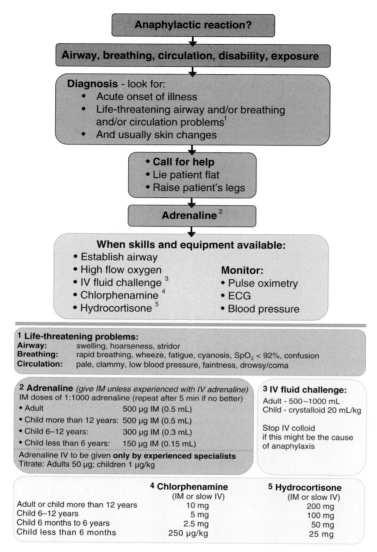

Figure 15.1 Anaphylaxis algorithm. (*Source*: Resuscitation Council UK, Resuscitation Guidelines 2005. Reproduced with kind permission of the Resuscitation Council UK.)

treat life-threatening problems as they present (Soar *et al.* 2008). The anaphylaxis algorithm (Figure 15.1) describes the key steps.

Immediate treatment (see Figure 15.1)

- All casualties should recline in a comfortable position. Lying flat with or without the legs elevated may be helpful if the casualty is hypotensive but unhelpful if there are breathing difficulties. Patients who are breathing and unconscious should be placed on their side (recovery position).

- The likely allergen should be removed if possible (i.e. stop drug infusion or blood transfusion).
- The highest concentration of oxygen available should be administered as soon as possible.
- Adrenaline is the most important drug for the treatment of anaphylactic reaction (McLean-Tooke *et al.* 2003). It reverses peripheral vasodilation and reduces oedema as well as dilating the bronchial airways, increasing the force of myocardial contraction and suppressing histamine and leukotriene release. Adrenaline seems to work best when given early after the onset of the reaction. Adverse effects are rare when the correct dose is given intramuscularly during anaphylaxis.
- The intramuscular (IM) route is the best for most individuals who have to give adrenaline to treat an anaphylactic reaction. The pulse, blood pressure, ECG and pulse oximetry should be monitored as soon as possible.
- For adults give an initial IM adrenaline dose of 0.5 mg (0.5 mL of 1:1000 adrenaline = 0.5 mg = 500 µg). Further doses can be given at 5-minute intervals according to the patient's response (see Chapter 12).
- Intravenous administration of adrenaline only applies to those experienced in the use and titration of vasopressors in their normal clinical practice.
- Autoinjectors are often given to patients at risk of anaphylaxis for their own use. At the time of writing, there are only two doses of adrenaline autoinjector commonly available: 0.15 and 0.3 mg. Healthcare professionals should be familiar with the use of the most commonly available autoinjector devices. If an adrenaline autoinjector is the only available adrenaline preparation when treating anaphylaxis, healthcare providers should use it.
- Give a rapid IV fluid challenge (500–1000 mL in adults) with further doses as necessary. Hartmann's solution or 0.9% saline are suitable fluids for initial resuscitation. Large volumes of fluid may leak from the patient's circulation during an anaphylactic reaction and this should be replaced as quickly as possible.
- Antihistamines are a second-line treatment for an anaphylactic reaction. An antihistamine (chlorphenamine) should be administered to block the effects of histamine release. The drug may cause hypotension. It must be given by either slow IV injection or IM injection. The adult dose is 10 mg IM or IV.
- Corticosteroids may help prevent or shorten protracted reactions. The dose of hydrocortisone for adults is 200 mg and must be given by slow IV or IM injection (Resuscitation Council UK 2008).
- Airway obstruction may develop rapidly if there is soft tissue swelling. It is important to consider early tracheal intubation and have the proper equipment readily available. A senior anaesthetist should also be involved as early as possible
- If the casualty is in cardiac arrest, CPR should be performed according to standard basic and advanced life support guidelines (refer to Chapters 6 and 7).

Further management
- Patients with a suspected anaphylactic reaction should be observed for at least 6 hours in a clinical area with facilities for treating life-threatening ABC problems. Patients should be warned of the possibility of an early recurrence of symptoms and in some circumstances be observed for up to 24 hours.

Discharge from hospital
- Patients should be given clear instructions to avoid contact with allergens and return to hospital if symptoms return.
- Consider giving antihistamines and oral steroid therapy for up to 3 days.
- **All patients** who have suffered a severe reaction should be referred to a specialist allergy clinic for further investigation and assessment.

ACUTE SEVERE ASTHMA
It is important to differentiate routine asthma care from that in acute severe asthma. This section will focus on acute or near-fatal asthma, a condition that is largely reversible; so, related deaths should be considered avoidable. Interventions are aimed at preventing respiratory and secondary cardiac arrest (Scottish Intercollegiate Guidelines Network (SIGN) and British Thoracic Society (BTS) 2003, Soar *et al.* 2005).

Most deaths related to acute severe asthma occur outside hospital. The contributing factors include:

- patients and their relatives seek medical care late because they do not understand or recognise the severity of the attack;
- emergency services or medical professionals may be slow to respond;
- patients with less severe asthma attacks may seek emergency care but after treatment they are discharged home and deteriorate further.

Cardiac arrest may occur in patients with severe asthma as a result of any of the following:

- hypoxia from mucus plugging or severe bronchospasm;
- cardiac arrhythmias from hypoxia or as a side-effect of beta-agonists and aminophylline;
- tension pneumothorax.

Recognising acute severe asthma
The ABCDE approach should be used to assess and treat patients. The following signs and symptoms may be present:

- wheezing is common; however, the severity does not correlate with the degree of airway obstruction;
- silent chest;
- cyanosis;
- weak or ineffective respiratory effort;
- fatigue, exhaustion, confusion or even coma;
- associated bradycardia and hypotension;
- arterial blood gases indicate hypoxia, acidaemia, normal or high carbon dioxide tension.

Responding to acute severe asthma

- All exacerbations of asthma must be treated aggressively to prevent near-fatal asthma and cardiac arrest. Patients should be cared for in a critical care environment with full monitoring and observation.
- Oxygen – high-flow oxygen (10–15 L/min) should be administered as soon as possible.
- First-line therapy – inhaled beta-agonists are recommended. Nebulised salbutamol, 5 mg in 5 mL of normal saline, should be administered with oxygen or alternatively 4–6 puffs through a metered dose inhaler with a holding chamber (SIGN and BTS 2003).
- Corticosteroid therapy – either oral or IV corticosteroids should be given in the first 30 minutes (SIGN and BTS 2003).
- Other therapies – inhaled anticholinergics, IV aminophylline, IV magnesium sulphate or Heliox may be used if patients fail to respond to other treatments (SIGN and BTS 2003).
- Fluid replacement – patients with severe acute asthma will often be dehydrated and benefit from IV fluid replacement.
- Basic and advanced life support – standard guidelines for basic and advanced life support should be followed.
- It may be difficult to ventilate the patient's lungs because of high airway resistance. Ventilation with a bag-valve-facemask may predispose the patient to gastric inflation. Tracheal intubation should be performed as early as possible.
- The patient may have a hyperinflated chest, making chest compressions difficult or impossible. To overcome this, allow a prolonged expiratory time between breaths (Soar et al. 2005).
- Any arrhythmias should be treated according to the current advanced life support (ALS) guidelines.

DROWNING

Drowning is defined as a process resulting in primary respiratory impairment from submersion or immersion in a liquid medium, usually water. This prevents the casualty from breathing air. The casualty may live or die after this process but whatever the outcome, the individual is involved in a drowning incident (Idris et al. 2003).

Recognising drowning

- Hypoxia and hypercarbia are important consequences of drowning. The outcome will largely depend on how long the patient was hypoxic. Therefore, oxygenation, ventilation and perfusion should be restored as rapidly as possible.
- Hypothermia may occur in water at 25°C or less and may be another factor to consider.
- Drowning is sometimes precipitated by an injury or medical condition. It is important to recognise and report this, if known. Examples may include (Idris et al. 2003):
  - seizure;

    ○ level of consciousness and/or motor function impaired by drugs, alcohol or hypothermia;

    ○ circulatory arrest (e.g. ventricular fibrillation (VF) or pulseless electrical activity);

    ○ trauma;

    ○ unconsciousness from any other cause.

Responding to drowning

- The ABCDE approach should be used to assess the casualty and resuscitation efforts should start at the scene if the casualty is to have the best chance of survival and full neurological recovery (Soar *et al.* 2005). Basic life support (BLS) should be commenced (refer to Chapter 6). It makes no difference if the accident is occurred in fresh or salt water.

- It is important to be aware of personal safety and minimise danger when reaching and recovering the casualty. Attempt to keep the casualty horizontal. Vertical removal from water may cause circulatory collapse (Soar *et al.* 2005).

- Resuscitation should start unless there are obvious lethal injuries, putrefaction or rigor mortis.

- If there is a possibility of spinal cord injury, such as after diving into shallow water, the spine should be immobilised during recovery. The jaw thrust should be used to open the airway, rather than head tilt, chin lift.

- Rescue breathing should begin as quickly as possible. It can be attempted once the rescuer can stand in the water or the casualty is on land. If it is difficult to perform mouth-to-mouth ventilation while supporting the casualty's head in the water, mouth-to-nose ventilation is an acceptable alternative.

- The airway should be inspected and any debris removed. It is **not** necessary to remove water from the airway before starting BLS. Attempting to tip the casualty head down will not help remove water and may cause vomiting and aspiration.

- Vomiting is a common occurrence in submersion events. The person's head should be turned to the side. Suction should be used to remove vomitus. Early tracheal intubation will help prevent aspiration of vomit.

- It may be difficult to palpate a pulse if the casualty is cold. If no signs of circulation are present, chest compressions should be started as soon as possible (ILCOR 2005). Do not attempt chest compressions while the casualty is still in water.

- Successful resuscitation with full neurological recovery has been reported in casualties with prolonged submersion in cold water; therefore, life support should continue for a longer period than usual (Soar *et al.* 2005).

Advanced life support

- ALS should be initiated without delay as necessary.

- Every drowning casualty should be transferred to a medical facility, even if only minimal resuscitation was necessary and the casualty regained consciousness. These patients are at high risk for developing other problems such as adult respiratory distress syndrome (ARDS), circulatory collapse or pulmonary oedema (Soar *et al.* 2005).

- The guidelines for hypothermia should be followed if the patient is hypothermic (<35°C).
- The insertion of a nasogastric tube will aid in decompressing and emptying the stomach.

ELECTROCUTION

Electrocution may occur as a result of domestic or industrial electricity or lightning strike. Adults are mostly likely to experience electrical injury in the workplace, while children are more at risk at home. There are approximately 1000 deaths worldwide every year from lightning strike (Auerbach 1995). Injuries may range from a transient, unpleasant sensation from contact with a low current to cardiac arrest from exposure to high voltage or current. The severity of electrical injury is also dependent on whether the current is alternating (a.c.) or direct (d.c.), magnitude of the energy delivered, resistance to current flow, pathway of current through the casualty and the area and duration of electrical contact (Lederer *et al.* 1999).

Recognising electrocution

- Contact with a.c. often causes tetanic contraction of skeletal muscle. Furthermore, casualties may not be able to release themselves from the source of electricity and respiratory arrest may also occur. The a.c. may also cause VF.
- Extensive tissue damage may occur along the electrical current pathway. A transthoracic (hand-to-hand) pathway is more likely to be fatal than a vertical (hand-to-foot) or straddle (foot-to-foot) pathway.
- Asystole or VF will most likely be present after a lightning strike as a result of a massive, direct shock that depolarises the entire myocardium. Respiratory muscle paralysis may also occur, leading to respiratory arrest. Secondary cardiac arrest may happen if respiratory arrest is not treated promptly and effectively.
- Immediately after any type of electrocution, the casualty may have respiratory or cardiac failure or both. The casualty may appear apnoeic or mottled or become unconscious. The casualty may also have contact burns at the point of entry and exit. It is essential to use the ABCDE approach in the initial assessment (refer to Chapter 3).

Responding to electrocution

- Safety – rescuers must be certain that they will not be in danger while attempting to rescue the casualty. Any power source should be turned off. Rescuers should also be aware of that a high-voltage electricity can 'arc' and conduct through the ground for up to a few metres around the casualty.
- Standard basic and advanced life support should be started as soon as possible.
- Airway – electrical burns around the face and neck may cause extensive soft tissue oedema that can lead to airway obstruction. Early intubation may be necessary. Head and spine trauma may also occur with electrocution. Spine immobilisation should be carried out until a thorough evaluation is made.
- Circulation – the commonest initial arrhythmia after high-voltage a.c. shock is VF. This may be due to the a.c. acting on the myocardium during the vulnerable

repolarisation phase, also known as R-on-T phenomenon (Lederer *et al.* 1999). This should be treated promptly with attempted defibrillation following standard protocols. Asystole is the commonest arrhythmia following high-voltage d.c. shock due to the massive d.c. that can depolarise the entire myocardium (Lederer *et al.* 1999). Treatment of asystole and any other arrhythmias should follow standard protocols (see Chapter 10).

- Other considerations – burns may occur from shoes or smouldering clothing. These items should be removed as soon as possible. Aggressive fluid therapy may also be required if there is serious tissue damage.
- Survivors of electrical injury should be monitored in hospital if they have a history of cardiorespiratory problems or have suffered loss of consciousness, cardiac arrest, ECG abnormalities or soft tissue damage and burns (Soar *et al.* 2005).

HYPOTHERMIA

Hypothermia occurs when the body core temperature falls below 35°C. It can happen when people with normal thermoregulation are exposed to cold environments or after immersion in cold water. In someone with impaired thermoregulation, hypothermia may occur from a mild cold insult. Hypothermia occurs in all four seasons and casualty presentation does not seem to depend only on ambient temperature (Soar *et al.* 2005).

Recognising hypothermia

- Clinical history and examination of the casualty may indicate hypothermia but it is confirmed by using a low-reading thermometer to measure core temperature (see Table 15.2). An oesophageal, rectal or tympanic thermometer should be used.
- Casualties may appear to be clinically dead because the brain and heart functions are slowed significantly and signs of life are very difficult to detect.
- Hypothermia can actually have a protective effect on the brain. Mild hypothermia may improve neurological function after a VF arrest (Nolan *et al.* 2003).
- Resuscitation should not be withheld based on clinical presentation. Also, once resuscitation attempts start, the team should continue until the casualties are rewarmed. This may mean a prolonged resuscitation.

Responding to hypothermia

- Preventing cardiac arrest – if the casualty is extremely cold but still has a perfusing rhythm, interventions should focus on assessment and support of

Table 15.2 Classification of hypothermia.

Classification of hypothermia	Temperature (°C)
Mild	35–32
Moderate	32–30
Severe	Below 30

airway, breathing and circulation, preventing further heat loss, rewarming and careful transport to a hospital.

- The casualty should be removed from the cold environment.
- Cold, wet clothing should be removed when it is practical. If the temperature is less than 25°C or there is wind, it may be better to leave wet garments on and wrap the casualty in blankets to avoid increased exposure (Auerbach 1995).
- Blankets and insulating equipment may be used to protect against further heat loss.
- Rough movement and activity can precipitate VF and should be avoided.
- Urgent procedures such as tracheal intubation or insertion of central venous catheters should be done gently and carefully while monitoring the heart rhythm closely.
- Core temperature and cardiac rhythm must be monitored.

Rewarming
- Casualties with a core temperature of less than 34°C should be rewarmed (Soar *et al.* 2005).
- Rewarming should occur at a rate that correlates with the rate of onset of hypothermia, although this may be difficult to determine (see Table 15.3).

Basic life support modifications
- BLS should be initiated according to the guidelines (described in Chapter 6).
- Hypothermia slows breathing and causes peripheral vasoconstriction. For this reason, breathing may be shallow and the pulse difficult to feel. It may be necessary to assess breathing and pulse for a longer period to confirm cardiac arrest (Soar *et al.* 2005). If the casualty is pulseless, start chest compressions immediately. If there is any doubt about whether the casualty has a pulse, it is better to commence chest compressions until experienced help arrives.
- The ventilation–compression ratio (30:2) should be the same as for casualties with a normal temperature. Hypothermia can make the chest wall feel stiff and

Table 15.3 Definitions of rewarming.

Passive rewarming	Achieved with blankets and a warm room. This method alone will not be effective for patients in cardiac arrest or severely hypothermic	All hypothermic patients
Active external warming	Heating devices (e.g. bair huggar), warm bath water or radiant heat. Use caution since some heating devices can cause tissue injury	Mild and moderate hypothermia
Active internal warming	Warmed, humidified oxygen, peritoneal, gastric, pleural or bladder lavage with warm fluid (40°C), intravenous administration of warmed fluids (e.g. normal saline). Follow local hospital policy	Severe hypothermia

ventilation and compressions more difficult. The lungs should be ventilated with enough volume to cause the chest to rise visibly. The rescuer should aim to achieve a compression depth of 4–5 cm.

- BLS should continue until the casualty is rewarmed.

Advanced life support modifications

- ALS should be initiated according to the ALS algorithm (see Chapter 7).
- Arrhythmias – procedures such as endotracheal intubation can cause VF. However, this should not be withheld when urgently indicated.
- Defibrillation – the hypothermic heart may be unresponsive to defibrillation. Continue CPR during this time (Soar *et al*. 2005).
- Drugs and drug administration – where possible, a central or large proximal vein should be cannulated. The casualty with hypothermia may not respond to cardioactive drugs. Drug metabolism is reduced and this may lead to a build-up of drugs in the system. Adrenaline and other drugs are generally withheld until the temperature is >30°C. Once this target is reached, the intervals between doses should be doubled and the lowest recommended dose given. Once the temperature is near normal, standard drug protocols can be used (Soar *et al*. 2005).

Death is not confirmed until the casualty is warm or attempts to raise core temperature are failed. A full recovery without neurological deficit may be possible even after prolonged hypothermic cardiac arrest (ILCOR 2005).

POISONING AND DRUG INTOXICATION

Poisoning is a leading cause of death in people less than 40 years old and is also the commonest cause of non-traumatic coma in this age group. Hospital admission is usually the result of self-poisoning with therapeutic or recreational drugs. Accidental poisoning is more common in children (Soar *et al*. 2005).

Recognising poisoning and drug intoxication

- Death is commonly caused by airway obstruction and respiratory arrest secondary to a decreased level of consciousness. Recognising airway and breathing problems should be a high priority.
- In an unconscious or arrested casualty, it may be difficult to determine whether the cause was poisoning. This must be excluded as a possible reason for the coma.

Responding to poisoning and drug intoxication

- The ABCDE approach should be used to assess and manage the casualty with poisoning while waiting for drug elimination from the body. Basic and advanced life support should proceed according to the standard guidelines when there is cardiac arrest (see Chapters 6 and 7).
- Airway and breathing – basic airway opening manoeuvres should be used. If the patient is not breathing, the lungs should be ventilated using a pocket mask or bag-valve-facemask and the highest possible concentration of oxygen. It is

especially important to avoid any mouth-to-mouth contact in the presence of toxins such as cyanide, hydrogen sulphide, corrosives and organophosphates (Resuscitation Council UK 2006).

- Early intubation – pulmonary aspiration of gastric contents is highly likely after poisoning. Early intubation is recommended in unconscious casualties who are unable to protect their own airway (Soar *et al.* 2005).
- It is important to identify the poison as soon as possible after resuscitation is started. Relatives, friends and emergency medical system crews may be able to provide information. The casualty should also be examined for needle puncture marks, tablet residues, signs of corrosion in the mouth or skin breakdown from lying in one position during prolonged coma.
- The TOXBASE (www.spib.axl.co.uk), co-ordinated by the Edinburgh Centre of the National Poisons Information Service (NPIS), can be accessed for specialist help on specific therapeutic measures.
- The emphasis with any poisoning should be on intensive supportive therapy, correction of hypoxia, acid–base and electrolyte disorders. The following specific therapeutic measures may be useful (Soar *et al.* 2005).
  - Gastric lavage is followed by activated charcoal – and is only recommended within one hour of ingesting the poison. Tracheal intubation should precede this intervention.
  - Haemodialysis or haemoperfusion may increase drug elimination.
  - Specific antidotes may be effective in certain situations, as shown in Table 15.4.

Table 15.4 A guide to poisons and possible antidotes or therapeutic measures.

Poison	Specific antidote or possible therapeutic measure
Paracetamol	N-acetylcysteine
Benzodiazapines (midazolam, diazepam, lorazepam)	Flumazenil
Tricyclic antidepressants	No specific antidote but administration of sodium bicarbonate may provide some myocardial protection and prevent arrhythmias
Opioids	Naloxone – the duration of action is shorter than the duration of most opioids and repeated doses may be needed
Cocaine toxicity	No specific antidote but small doses of intravenous benzodiazepines are effective first-line agents. Nitrates may be used as second-line therapy for myocardial ischaemia. Labetalol (alpha- and beta-blocker) is helpful for tachycardia and hypertensive emergencies
Digoxin	Digoxin-specific Fab antibodies (Digi-bind)
Organophosphate insecticides	High-dose atropine
Cyanide	Sodium nitrite, sodium thiosulphate or dicobalt edetate

PREGNANCY

Pregnancy creates a unique situation because there are two people to resuscitate. The emphasis must be on effective life support for the mother and this will in turn optimise fetal outcome. There may be many different reasons for cardiac arrest in pregnant women and it is most commonly related to changes and events that occur around the time of delivery (Soar *et al.* 2005).

Recognising an emergency in pregnancy

Causes of maternal cardiac arrest may include haemorrhage, pulmonary embolism, amniotic fluid embolism, placental abruption, eclampsia and drug toxicity. Physiological changes occur during pregnancy and these must be considered during an emergency. Use the ABCDE approach when assessing the casualty.

- Gastric emptying is delayed after the first trimester of pregnancy and there may be an increased risk of pulmonary aspiration of gastric contents.
- Anatomical changes such as breast enlargement, obesity of the neck and glottic oedema may make airway management difficult. Also, in later stages of pregnancy, the diaphragm is splinted by a large uterus and higher than normal inflation pressures may be needed to achieve effective ventilation.
- Cardiovascular problems may occur because the uterus presses down against the inferior vena cava and reduces or blocks blood flow to the heart.

Responding

- An obstetrician and a neonatologist should be involved as early as possible (Resuscitation Council UK 2006).
- All principles of basic and advanced life support apply to the pregnant woman.
- Cardiac arrest may be prevented with early intervention. Cardiac output and venous return may be improved by relieving pressure on the inferior vena cava and aorta (Soar *et al.* 2005). This can be achieved by:
  - placing sandbags, pillows or a purpose-made (Cardiff) wedge under the patient's right buttock and lower back;
  - placing the patient in the left lateral position;
  - manually moving the uterus to the left.
- Chest compression is performed in the standard way. The rescuer should be aware of that it may be more difficult because of the breast hypertrophy and splinting of the diaphragm.
- Arrhythmias should be treated according to standard protocols.

Emergency caesarean section is recommended after five minutes of unsuccessful resuscitation to improve the chances of both fetal and maternal survival (Resuscitation Council UK 2006).

REVIEW OF LEARNING

- ❏ Special circumstances may occur that require the team to modify its approach to resuscitation.
- ❏ Recognising and responding early may prevent cardiac arrest in special circumstances.

❏ Anaphylaxis is increasingly common. Epinephrine (adrenaline) given intra-muscularly is considered the most important drug for any severe anaphylactic reaction.

❏ Acute severe asthma is largely reversible and related deaths should be considered avoidable.

❏ Asthma exacerbations must be treated aggressively with oxygen, inhaled beta-agonists and corticosteroid therapy.

❏ Hypoxia and hypercarbia are consequences of drowning. Oxygenation, ventilation and perfusion should be restored as rapidly as possible.

❏ Successful resuscitation with full neurological recovery has been reported in casualties with prolonged submersion in cold water; therefore, life support should continue for a longer period than usual.

❏ Electrocution may occur from an a.c. or d.c. Asystole and VF are common arrhythmias that should be treated according to the universal algorithm.

❏ Mild hypothermia may improve neurological function after a VF arrest.

❏ Rewarming the hypothermic casualty should occur at a rate that correlates with the rate of onset of hypothermia.

❏ Death in poisoning is commonly caused by airway obstruction and respiratory arrest secondary to a decreased level of consciousness. Recognising airway and breathing problems should be a high priority.

❏ Pregnancy creates a unique situation because there are two people to resuscitate. The emphasis must be on effective life support for the mother and this will in turn optimise fetal outcome.

❏ Cardiac output and venous return may be improved by relieving pressure on the inferior vena cava and aorta in the pregnant casualty.

Case study

Fred Hughes is a 70-year-old man admitted to the hospital for treatment of community-acquired pneumonia. A few minutes after the first dose of IV benzylpenicillin, Fred complains of feeling sick, vomits and becomes unresponsive.

What do you suspect is happening? What other signs and symptoms might be present?

It is likely that Mr Hughes is having an anaphylactic reaction due to the administration of IV antibiotic. Specific signs and symptoms to watch out for include varying degrees of angio-oedema, urticaria, dyspnoea and hypotension. The patient may also have rhinitis, conjunctivitis, diarrhoea and a sense of impending doom. The skin colour often changes and the patient may appear either flushed or pale. Cardiovascular collapse is caused by vasodilation and loss of plasma from the blood compartment into the tissues. It is a common clinical manifestation, especially in response to IV drugs or stings.

During your physical examination you note that Fred's skin is red and flushed and there is generalised urticaria. His tongue is swollen and he is having difficulty breathing. His heart rate is 120 bpm and his blood pressure is 65/40.

How would you respond to this situation?

- Call for help.
- Stop the infusion of benzylpenicillin.
- Administer high-flow oxygen (10–15 L/min). Assess the patient for airway obstruction and be prepared with airway adjuncts as discussed in Chapter 7.
- Give adrenaline 1:1000 solution of 0.5 mL intramuscularly. Alternatively, use an Epipen.
- Adrenaline IM may be repeated after about five minutes if there is no clinical improvement or if the patient deteriorates after the initial treatment, especially if hypotension causes the level of consciousness to become or remain impaired.
- Give a rapid IV fluid challenge – 500–1000 mL of Hartmann's solution or 0.9% saline.
- Administer an antihistamine (chlorphenamine). It must be given either by slow IV injection or by IM injection. The dose for an adult is 10 mg.
- Consider administration of hydrocortisone 200 mg slowly IV or IM.

REFERENCES

Auerbach, P.S. (ed) (1995) *Wilderness Medicine: Management of Wilderness and Environmental Emergencies*, 3rd edn. Mosby, Philadelphia.

Idris, A.H., Berg, R.A., Bierens, J. *et al.* (2003) Recommended guidelines for uniform reporting of data from drowning: the 'Utstein Style'. *Resuscitation* **59**, 45–57.

International Liaison Committee on Resuscitation (2005) International consensus on cardiopulmonary resuscitation and emergency cardiovascular care science with treatment recommendations. Part 4. Advanced life support. *Resuscitation* **67**, 213–47.

Lederer, W., Wiedermann, F.J., Cerchiari, E. & Baubin, M.A. (1999) Electricity-associated injuries. I: outdoor management of current-induced casualties. *Resuscitation* **43**, 69–77.

McLean-Tooke, A.P., Bethune, C.A., Fay, A.C. & Spickett, G.P. (2003) Adrenaline in the treatment of anaphylaxis: what is the evidence? *BMJ* **327**, 1332–5.

Nolan, J.P., Morley, P.T., Vanden Hoek, T.L. & Hickey, R.W., for the ALS Task Force (2003) Therapeutic hypothermia after cardiac arrest. An advisory statement by the Advanced Life Support Task Force of the International Liaison Committee on Resuscitation. *Resuscitation* **57**, 231–5.

Resuscitation Council UK (2006) *Advanced Life Support Course Provider Manual*, 5th edn. Resuscitation Council UK, London.

Resuscitation Council UK (2008) *Emergency Treatment of Anaphylactic Reactions: Guidelines for Healthcare Providers*. Available online at: www.resus.org.uk.

Scottish Intercollegiate Guidelines Network and British Thoracic Society (2003) *British Guideline on the Management of Asthma*. Available online at: www.brit-thoracic.org.uk/sign.

Soar, J., Deakin C.D., Nolan, J.P. *et al.* (2005) European Resuscitation Council guidelines for resuscitation 2005. Section 7. Cardiac arrest in special circumstances. *Resuscitation* **67** (suppl I), 135–70.

Soar, J., Pumphrey, R., Cant, A. *et al.* (2008) Emergency treatment of anaphylactic reactions – Guidelines for healthcare providers. *Resuscitation* **77**, 157–69.

Resuscitation of the Seriously Injured Casualty

16

Jas Soar

INTRODUCTION

Trauma is the major cause of morbidity and mortality in otherwise healthy adults, with 3000 people dying and 30 000 being injured every day on the world's roads. Trauma is the leading cause of death in the first three decades of life and millions are injured each year and survive. For many, the injury causes temporary pain and inconvenience but for some it leads to disability, chronic pain and a profound change in lifestyle. Preventive public health measures such as safety belts and health and safety laws are the key to decreasing these numbers.

Trauma deaths occur in three peaks.

- Peak 1 refers to 'immediate' deaths at the scene of an accident due to lethal and usually untreatable injuries.
- Peak 2 describes deaths occurring in the first few hours after injury. These early deaths are usually due to airway, breathing and circulation failure or head injury. They may be prevented by early treatment during what is called the *golden hour* of trauma resuscitation.
- Peak 3 deaths occur weeks or months after the injury. These late deaths usually occur in the critical care unit and are due to sepsis and multiple organ failure.

AIMS

This chapter provides a structured approach to the initial resuscitation of the seriously injured casualty.

LEARNING OUTCOMES

At the end of the chapter, the reader will be able to:

- ❏ prepare for *reception* of the seriously injured casualty;
- ❏ understand the *role of the trauma team*;
- ❏ understand the *key steps in the initial management* of the seriously injured casualty;
- ❏ safely *transfer the casualty* for definitive care.

RECEPTION OF THE SERIOUSLY INJURED CASUALTY

The ambulance service will often warn the emergency department of the arrival of a seriously injured casualty. This allows preparation of the resuscitation room

> **Box 16.1 Factors associated with serious injury.**
>
> Fall from a height of 4 m or more than 4 m
> High-speed impact in road traffic accident
> Death of other passengers at scene of road accident
> Ejection from vehicle
> Motorcyclist with no helmet involved in accident
> Significant damage to the passenger compartment of vehicle

and alerting of the trauma team. However, there will always be casualties who arrive unexpectedly with serious injury and therefore the emergency department should be prepared to receive casualties at short notice.

The resuscitation room

The resuscitation room needs to be ready to accept casualties. Drugs and equipment stocks should be checked at the beginning of every shift, using a checklist to ensure items are not missed. Equipment such as defibrillators, oxygen cylinders and suction should be in working order.

THE TRAUMA TEAM

Trauma team members should be ready in the resuscitation room to receive the seriously injured casualty (Gwinnutt & Driscoll 2003). Information received from ambulance control will usually indicate whether the trauma team is required and Box 16.1 lists factors associated with serious injuries. There should be a medical and nursing team leader and the team should include members with the following skills:

- assessment and treatment of the seriously injured;
- advanced airway skills – this includes the ability to perform a rapid-sequence induction (RSI) and tracheal intubation;
- advanced cannulation skills;
- radiographer for X-ray images;
- portering;
- record and timekeeping;
- team member for liaising with relatives or to accompany relatives if they wish to be present during the resuscitation.

Personal protective equipment

Trauma team members need to ensure their personal safety by taking universal precautions. Minimum precautions when dealing with a seriously injured casualty include:

- eye protection;
- gloves;
- waterproof aprons;
- X-ray gowns.

All body fluids should be treated as potentially infected. When casualties arrive in the emergency department, they will often be dressed and covered in debris that can include glass fragments and other sharp objects and extra precautions are needed for casualties of biological or chemical attack. These casualties require decontamination at the scene of the incident or immediately on arrival to hospital prior to entering the emergency department.

IN-HOSPITAL RESUSCITATION

Successful resuscitation of the seriously injured casualty requires a systematic approach to patient management. The most commonly used system is based on advanced trauma life support course principles developed by the American College of Surgeons in the 1970s (American College of Surgeons 1997). Team members perform a number of tasks simultaneously, with the initial management consisting of three phases:

- primary survey and resuscitation;
- secondary survey;
- definitive care.

Primary survey and resuscitation

The primary survey identifies and treats life-threatening injuries in the order in which they are most likely to kill the patient. The priorities for recognising and responding are:

- *A*: airway with cervical spine control;
- *B*: breathing;
- *C*: circulation and haemorrhage control;
- *D*: dysfunction, refers to neurological status;
- *E*: exposure and environment.

A: airway and cervical spine

It is important that the casualty has a clear airway and adequate oxygenation. The airway is assessed and managed as described in Chapter 9, with the proviso that the cervical spine is protected. A patient who can speak clearly has a clear airway, whereas the unconscious patient may require help with maintaining an open airway and breathing. Snoring, gurgling and stridor can indicate an upper airway obstruction.

A cervical spine injury should be assumed in all patients with severe trauma until it has been excluded. Jaw thrust and airway adjuncts are the preferred methods to open the airway of the unconscious trauma patient.

The cervical spine is immobilised with one of two methods:

- manual in-line stabilisation: a team member holds the casualty's head and neck in the neutral position;
- semi-rigid cervical collar blocks and tape (see Figure 16.1).

Seriously injured patients are at high risk of vomiting and aspiration of gastric contents. Patients with a decreased conscious level and inability to protect their airway require early tracheal intubation which is ideally performed

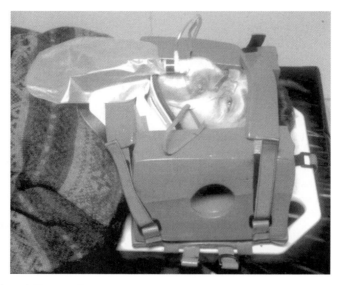

Figure 16.1 Immobilisation of the cervical spine using collar blocks and straps.

using an RSI technique. This requires administration of an intravenous sedative, a fast-onset, short-acting muscle relaxant (suxamethonium) and the application of cricoid pressure. Once the patient is fully sedated and relaxed the trachea is intubated. This requires specialist training (Clancy & Nolan 2002). The head is held using manual in-line stabilisation during tracheal intubation to ensure the cervical spine is not moved. This is preferable to using head blocks and a cervical collar, which can make access and mouth opening difficult.

B: breathing

All patients must initially be given oxygen at the highest concentration possible. A fully conscious patient who is breathing normally requires a facemask with reservoir and high-flow oxygen (10–15 L/min). A patient who is not breathing will require assistance with breathing using a bag-valve-mask device.

Chest injuries will cause difficulty in breathing and the patient may have a fast or slow respiratory rate and also be hypoxic. The need for oxygen to maintain a normal oxygen saturation also indicates that there is a problem. The team leader should look for and treat life-threatening chest injuries in the primary survey. These can be diagnosed clinically and excluded in the primary survey (see Table 16.1). The recognition of and response to these injuries require specialist training.

C: circulation

'Shock' is defined as inadequate organ perfusion and tissue oxygenation. The recognition of hypovolaemic shock is based on clinical findings: hypotension, tachycardia, tachypnoea, altered conscious level as well as hypothermia, pallor, cool extremities, decreased capillary refill and decreased urine production.

Table 16.1 Chest injuries identified and treated in the primary survey.

Injury	Recognition	Response
Tension pneumothorax	Decreased air entry, decreased expansion and hyperresonance to percussion on the side of injury Trachea deviated away from injured side	Needle thoracocentesis. A large-bore needle is placed in the second intercostal space, midclavicular line to relieve the tension. A chest drain is then inserted
Open pneumothorax	There is a hole in the casualty's chest wall, which sucks on inspiration: 'sucking chest wound'	The hole should be covered with a square waterproof dressing that is taped down on three sides. This stops air being sucked in but allows air to escape through the hole. A chest drain is then inserted
Massive haemothorax	There is bleeding in the chest. The affected side will have decreased expansion and air entry and will be dull to percussion. A large volume of blood can be lost in the chest so the patient may be shocked	Chest drain inserted on injured side. If there is a large amount of blood loss the patient requires immediate surgery to stop the bleeding
Flail chest	This occurs when there are a large number of rib fractures. A portion of the chest wall (flail segment) moves freely. This limits expansion of the lungs on inspiration. The flail segment will not move on chest expansion. The extent of the rib fractures also indicates that the chest has been struck with a large force so there is usually an underlying lung injury (lung contusion)	Oxygen, analgesia to make breathing less painful. Tracheal intubation and controlled ventilation if there is severe lung contusion
Cardiac tamponade	Bleeding around the heart may prevent it pumping effectively. It can occur after blunt or penetrating trauma. The patient will be shocked (low blood pressure) and there may be a wound (between the nipples or shoulder blades). There may be muffled heart sounds and distended neck veins	Pericardiocentesis. A drain is inserted into the pericardial space and any blood around the heart removed. Effective treatment may require an urgent thoracotomy in the emergency room (Rhee et al. 2000)

A low blood pressure (hypotension) is assumed to be due to bleeding (haemorrhage) in the injured patient unless proven otherwise. The amount of blood loss after trauma is often poorly assessed and in blunt trauma is usually underestimated. Often large volumes of blood may be hidden in the abdominal and chest cavity. A femoral fracture can be associated with a 2 L blood loss. This is a large proportion of the blood volume if one considers that the total blood volume of a 70 kg male is 5 L. Bleeding must therefore be identified and stopped to prevent hypovolaemic shock. Hypovolaemic shock in the adult can be categorised into four stages (I, II, III and IV) based on the amount of blood loss (see Table 16.2).

Table 16.2 Categories of hypovolaemic shock.

	I	II	III	IV
Blood loss (L)	<0.75	0.75–1.5	1.5–2.0	>2.0
Percentage blood loss (%)	<15	15–30	30–40	>40
Heart rate	<100	>100	>120	>140 or low
Systolic BP	Normal	Normal	Decreased	Decreased++
Diastolic BP	Normal	Raised	Decreased	Decreased++
Pulse pressure	Normal	Decreased	Decreased	Decreased
Capillary refill	Normal	Delayed	Delayed	Delayed
Skin colour	Normal	Pale	Very pale	Very pale/cold
Respiratory rate	14–20	20–30	30–40	>35 or low
Mental state	Normal/ anxious	Anxious	Anxious/ confused	Confused/ drowsy
Fluid choice	None/ crystalloid	Crystalloid/ colloid	Blood	Blood

Pulse pressure = systolic BP – diastolic BP

Capillary refill is measured by pressing a distal digit at heart level for five seconds. A normal capillary return time is less than two seconds. This can be affected by cold weather so it must be interpreted with other signs and symptoms.

The response to hypovolaemic shock is to stop the bleeding and correct the blood volume. Wound bleeding be stopped by applying direct pressure. Internal blood loss may require rapid transfer to an operating theatre for surgical control of blood loss. Blood volume is restored using intravenous fluids and blood.

Intravenous access must be established early during the resuscitation. Two large-bore cannulae (14 gauge) should be inserted. At this time blood should be taken for the following investigations:

- full blood count;
- urea and electrolytes;
- coagulation study;
- glucose;
- cross-matching;
- consider a pregnancy test in females of childbearing age;
- arterial blood gases.

It is pointless giving large amounts of intravenous fluids to a patient who is actively bleeding if no effort is made to stop the blood loss. The role of fluid resuscitation at this stage is to keep the patient alive until there is definitive control of bleeding. As mentioned previously, this requires direct pressure, splinting of fractures or immediate surgery. Failure to stop bleeding results in excessive fluid administration. This can cause increased blood loss as clots may be disrupted at the injury site due to increased blood pressure and dilution of clotting factors and platelets (Revell *et al.* 2003).

The choice of resuscitation fluids is controversial (Nolan 2001). Fluids that could be used include crystalloids (Hartmann's or 0.9% normal saline) and colloids such as gelatins (Gelofusin, Haemaccel), dextrans or starches. Current evidence indicates that there is no real advantage in using the more expensive colloids over cheaper crystalloids for initial fluid management in trauma patients. The volume given should be based on the response in terms of improvements in blood pressure, pulse and conscious level.

The amount and urgency of blood transfusion will depend on the degree of hypovolaemia. In multiple injuries, it may be necessary to order 6–10 units of blood. If blood is required immediately, the blood bank will supply group O blood, which has not been grouped or cross-matched to the patient. If it is possible to wait for 10–15 minutes, the blood bank can supply group-confirmed blood. This is the same blood group as the patient but has not been cross-matched with the patient's blood. Fully grouped and cross-matched blood takes much longer to process.

All fluids and blood products should be warmed before infusion. Critically ill patients tolerate lower haemoglobin concentrations than previously thought. During resuscitation, a haemoglobin concentration of between 7 and 9 g/dL (normal range approximately 12–16 g/dL) is likely to be adequate, with the possible exception of those patients with acute myocardial infarction and unstable angina (Hebert *et al.* 1999).

If cardiac arrest occurs resuscitation should follow ALS guidelines as described in Chapter 7. Special attention should be paid to stopping blood loss and restoring the circulating volume. If cardiac arrest is associated with a penetrating chest wound, an emergency thoracotomy at the scene may be lifesaving (Rhee *et al.* 2000). Cardiac arrest associated with trauma has a poor prognosis (Hopson *et al.* 2003).

D: disability

Disability refers to the casualty's neurological status. The following need to be assessed.

- Conscious level is assessed quickly using the AVPU method (see below). The Glasgow Coma Scale (GCS) score is the preferred method for assessing conscious level (see Table 16.3). A scoring chart should be available on the resuscitation room wall. The best score is recorded. Some patients who appear deeply unconscious may respond to a painful stimulus. The lowest score that can be achieved is 3. Patients with a GCS score less than 8 are in a coma and will usually require tracheal intubation. Common causes of a low GCS score in the trauma casualty are hypovolaemia, hypoxia, head injury and drugs or alcohol.
- Pupillary reflexes – both pupils need to be assessed simultaneously. They should be equal in size. Both pupils should react when a light is shone on one eye (direct and consensual light reflex present).
- Lateralising signs – the patient should move both sides of their body.

AVPU for assessing conscious level:

A – Alert. The casualty is awake and fully orientated.
V – Vocalising. The casualty is awake and confused.

Table 16.3 Glasgow Coma Scale.

Eyes	
Open spontaneously	4
Open to speech	3
Open to pain	2
None	1
Verbal	
Orientated	5
Confused	4
Inappropriate words	3
Incomprehensible sounds	2
None	1
Motor	
Obeys commands	6
Localises pain	5
Withdraws from pain	4
Flexion to pain	3
Extension to pain	2
None	1

P – Pain. The casualty only responds to a painful stimulus, such as pressure on the nail bed or supraorbital ridge.

U – Unresponsive. There is no response to painful stimuli.

If a head injury is suspected, the casualty's ABCs need to be optimised as described above to prevent further brain damage. This requires tracheal intubation with sedation and controlled ventilation if the GCS score is 8 or less. Further care needs to be discussed with a neurosurgeon. The response will include a CT scan and possible transfer to a neurosurgical centre for further management. Hypoxia and hypotension must be avoided to improve outcome in severe head injury (Chestnut *et al*. 1993). Current national guidelines for management of head injury should be followed (Scottish Intercollegiate Guidelines Network (SIGN) 2000).

Large numbers of casualties present with minor head injuries and concussion. Departments usually have guidelines to deal with these with regards to investigations (X-rays, CT scans) and admission or discharge. Those discharged after head injuries need to be supervised by a responsible adult and advised to return to the department if symptoms (including headache, blurred vision, nausea, vomiting) worsen. A head injury advice sheet with emergency contact details should be provided. Neurological status can change over time. Assessments need to be taken and recorded at regular intervals and recorded on a 'Neurological Observation' chart.

E: exposure and environment

The casualty must be adequately exposed to allow a full head-to-toe assessment, requiring the removal of their clothes. Specially designed cutters are available to assist in this. Patient's dignity must be maintained at all times. Efforts should be made to prevent hypothermia although a mild degree of hypothermia may be beneficial in head injury patients (Bernard & Buist 2003). It is therefore important not to over warm patients. The patient's temperature should be measured regularly and controlled appropriately.

Monitoring

Monitoring of the patient is required during resuscitation. The most important monitors are the members of the resuscitation team who look, listen and interact with the patient. The use of monitoring equipment allows earlier detection and measurement of physiological variables such as pulse, heart rate and blood pressure. A monitor will not tell you that the patient is bleeding or has a tension pneumothorax. It will merely alert you to any changes in physiological variables that occur with these conditions. The minimum monitoring required for the seriously injured patient includes:

- pulse rate and oxygen saturation using a pulse oximeter;
- blood pressure using an automated cuff;
- electrocardiogram will give you the heart rate and rhythm;
- respiratory rate;
- capnography to measure end-tidal carbon dioxide concentration in the intubated ventilated patient;
- temperature monitoring – tympanic temperature probes are most commonly used to measure temperature intermittently. An oesophageal probe is best for continuous monitoring in the intubated and ventilated patient.

The record-keeper should enter these details on the trauma observation chart. For an example of a trauma chart, see: www.emergency-nurse.com/tchart/.

History of events

It is important that the cause of the injury is known and the exact sequence of events gives an idea of what type of injuries to expect. The mnemonic AMPLE offers a useful way of remembering the important areas of the history:

- A – allergies;
- M – medications;
- P – past medical history;
- L – last meal;
- E – events.

It is important to ensure that all the information required is obtained before paramedics or relatives leave the emergency department. It is also vital to correctly identify the casualty and affix name bands.

Adjuncts to the primary survey

To complete the primary survey of the seriously injured casualty, the following must also be considered.

- X-rays – chest and pelvic X-rays are a mandatory part of the primary survey in the seriously injured casualty. These can be taken whilst resuscitation is ongoing. Imaging for spinal fractures can wait until the patient is stabilised as long as precautions are taken to immobilise the spine. Time should not be wasted obtaining cervical spine images if this will delay treatment for life-threatening injuries.

- Nasogastric tube insertion – if the patient has a base-of-skull fracture, the nasal route should be avoided.
- Urinary catheter insertion – expert help is needed if there is a pelvic fracture or evidence of urethral injury.
- Analgesia is an important part of initial treatment. Small doses of intravenous morphine can be titrated to relieve pain. Reducing fractures also reduces pain.
- There is a high risk of pressure sores developing if an injured casualty is immobilised on a long spine board. It is therefore good practice to remove the board as early as possible (Porter & Allison 2003). This requires log rolling the patient (see below).
- Further management of the seriously injured casualty often requires the involvement of a number of specialists (e.g. orthopaedic surgeons, neurosurgeons, radiologists and intensivists). It is important to contact them early if their services are likely to be required.

Secondary survey

As soon as it is confirmed that the casualty is not going to die from an immediately life-threatening injury, the secondary survey can commence. The secondary survey is a top-to-toe, thorough front-and-back assessment of the patient and it identifies injuries that are not immediately life threatening. In some patients, this will mean that the secondary survey takes place after emergency surgery for traumatic haemorrhage.

It is important to constantly review the patient during initial resuscitation. If the patient's condition deteriorates, he or she should be reassessed starting at the beginning of the primary survey with airway and cervical spine.

The log roll (see Figure 16.2)

The log roll allows assessment of the casualty's back. The procedure requires four helpers to roll the patient (one at the head and three along the sides of the casualty) and one person to examine the casualty. The person at the head maintains manual in-line stabilisation of the head and neck. The spine should be kept in alignment during the roll. The three team members on the side position themselves so one member is at the chest, one at the abdomen/pelvis and one at the legs. These three team members reach across the casualty to the opposite side of their body and place their hands on the casualty in preparation to log roll. On direction from the person at the head, the command is given to roll the casualty on the 'count of three'. The casualty is rolled towards the three team members and the back is inspected in detail and all clothing, straps and debris removed. The spine is palpated and the lungs auscultated. The rectum is examined to check for perineal injuries and anal tone. This is also a good time to remove the long spine board, as it is uncomfortable to lie on and can cause pressure sore development.

When the examination is complete, the process is reversed and the casualty is rolled onto their back in a controlled manner, keeping the spine aligned.

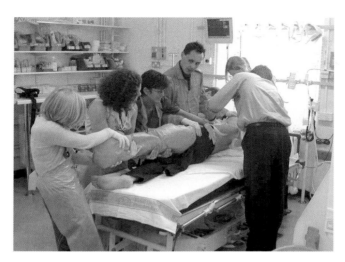

Figure 16.2 The trauma team log rolling a casualty.

Transfer and definitive care

Definitive care of the seriously injured casualty requires transfer to an operating theatre or intensive care unit, often via the radiology department for scans. This may require transfer to another hospital. Safe transfer requires:

- A stable patient – this is not always possible. If a patient is hypovolaemic from a ruptured spleen rapid transfer to an operating theatre and immediate surgery is needed to stop the bleeding.
- Trained personnel to monitor and manage changes in the patient's condition during transfer.
- Communication – the receiving hospital or department should know that patient is coming. Copies of notes, X-rays and any cross-matched blood should accompany the patient.
- Monitoring equipment – the same monitoring as used in the initial management of the patient is continued during transfer. This requires robust, portable lightweight monitors with adequate battery life.
- Oxygen and supplies – there should be enough oxygen in the cylinders and drug and fluid supplies to complete the journey.

Finally, the tetanus immunity status of the casualty should be checked. If there is no history available, the casualty should be considered unimmunised. Antibiotic therapy needs to be started in those with wounds and injuries where there is a high risk of infection.

REVIEW OF LEARNING

❏ Trauma is a major cause of morbidity and mortality in children and young adults.
❏ Trauma care requires a multiprofessional team approach.
❏ The primary survey recognises life-threatening 'ABCD' problems.

❏ A rapid response to immediate life-threatening problems saves lives.
❏ The top-to-toe secondary survey ensures that no injuries are missed.
❏ The patient requires safe transfer for definitive care.

Case study

You are rostered to work in the emergency department resuscitation room. Ambulance control has informed the department that a casualty with multiple injuries will be arriving in approximately ten minutes.

What preparations need to be made?

Members of the trauma team need to be alerted. The resuscitation room should always be ready to receive seriously injured patients. Team leaders should allocate tasks. Team members should don protective clothing.

A young female casualty arrives in the resuscitation room. She appears to be unconscious and looks extremely pale. She is snoring and breathing very fast. The left side of the chest is not moving. There is decreased air entry on the left side and it is hyper-resonant on percussion. Her right thigh looks swollen and deformed. The ambulance crew have already immobilised the casualty on a long spine board. She is wearing a cervical collar and her head is strapped between blocks. She is receiving oxygen.

What are the priorities in the care of the injured casualty?

A primary survey is performed using an ABCD approach. Life-threatening injuries are treated as they are identified.

- Airway with cervical spine control – the casualty is snoring. A jaw thrust is performed to avoid moving the cervical spine. The cervical spine is already immobilised using blocks and a hard collar (see Figure 16.1). High-flow oxygen is administered.
- Breathing – the patient is breathing very fast and has signs and symptoms of a left tension pneumothorax (see Table 16.1). This is treated by inserting a cannula in the left second intercostal space in the midclavicular line. This relives the tension pneumothorax. The circulation is assessed whilst preparing equipment to insert a chest drain on the left side.

The casualty's circulation is assessed and monitoring attached. She is very pale and has cool peripheries with a capillary refill time of three seconds. The paramedics have informed the team that her name is Penelope and that she fell off her horse. You are recording the observations: respiratory rate 30 breaths/min, oxygen saturation 97% on 15 L/min oxygen, pulse 130 bpm, blood pressure 80/40 mm Hg.

Can you explain these observations and what is the initial management?

Penelope has shock which is most likely to be due to bleeding causing hypovolaemia (see Table 16.2). The initial management includes obtaining intravenous access, sending blood for investigations, giving intravenous fluids and stopping any bleeding. There is an obvious right femoral fracture that could explain some of the blood loss.

The radiographer has taken chest and pelvic X-rays whilst resuscitation is ongoing. The chest drain has been inserted and can be seen on the chest X-ray. The pelvic X-ray shows a complex fracture which would explain the severity of the shock.

The orthopaedic surgeons stabilise the pelvic and femoral fractures in the resuscitation room as this will hopefully stop bleeding. The pelvic fracture is stabilised by applying an external fixator and the femoral fracture using a traction splint. Intravenous fluids (2000 mL warmed Hartmann's) are given to correct the circulating volume and Penelope's observations are now: pulse 110 bpm, blood pressure 90/50 mm Hg. Penelope now seems to be moaning. You have been asked to assess and monitor her neurological status.

What observations will you make?

You need to assess her neurological status, whether using the GCS score. It is important to check whether she is moving all four limbs and that her pupils are normal.

Penelope may have a spinal injury and her back needs to be examined.

How are we going to achieve this without further harming her and injuring ourselves?

We need to log roll Penelope to assess her spine. We first explain to Penelope what we are going to do. The technique used for the log roll is described above and in Figure 16.2.

Once Penelope has been stabilised in the resuscitation room, she is transferred to the radiology department for further imaging studies. She is then taken to the high dependency unit. Later that evening she has successful surgery to fix her fractures. She spends four days on the high dependency unit and a further five weeks in hospital recovering from her injuries. Six months later, she is still having physiotherapy. She has missed her final term at university and is not working. Her accident has had a long-term impact on her social, psychological and physical well-being.

CONCLUSION

The initial response to resuscitating the seriously injured casualty requires prior preparation and a team approach. Early effective management may prevent death in those seriously injured patients who survive to reach hospital.

REFERENCES

American College of Surgeons (1997) *Advanced Trauma Life Support Manual*. American College of Surgeons, Chicago.

Bernard, S.A. & Buist, M. (2003) Induced hypothermia in critical care medicine: a review. *Critical Care Medicine* **31** (7), 2041–51.

Chestnut, R.M., Marshall, L.F., Klauber, M.R. *et al.* (1993) The role of secondary brain injury in determining outcome from severe head injury. *Journal of Trauma* **34** (2), 216–22.

Clancy, M. & Nolan, J. (2002) Airway management in the emergency department. *Emergency Medical Journal* **19** (1), 2–3.

Gwinnutt, C. & Driscoll, P. (2003) *Trauma Resuscitation. The Team Approach*, 2nd edn. Bios, Oxford.

Hebert, P.C., Wells, G., Blajchman, M.A. *et al.*, for Transfusion Requirements in Critical Care Investigators, Canadian Critical Care Trials Group (1999) A multicenter, randomized, controlled clinical trial of transfusion requirements in critical care. *New England Journal of Medicine* **340** (6), 409–17.

Hopson, L.R., Hirsh, E., Delgado, J. *et al.*, for National Association of EMS Physicians, American College of Surgeons Committee on Trauma (2003) Guidelines for withholding or termination of resuscitation in prehospital traumatic cardiopulmonary arrest: joint position statement of the National Association of EMS Physicians and the American College of Surgeons Committee on Trauma. *Journal of the American College of Surgeons* **196** (1), 106–12.

Nolan, J. (2001) Fluid resuscitation for the trauma patient. *Resuscitation* **48** (1), 57–69.

Porter, K.M. & Allison, K.P. (2003) The UK emergency department practice for spinal board unloading. Is there conformity? *Resuscitation* **58** (1), 117–20.

Revell, M., Greaves, I. & Porter, K. (2003) Endpoints for fluid resuscitation in hemorrhagic shock. *Trauma* **54** (5, suppl), S63–7.

Rhee, P.M., Acosta, J., Bridgeman, A., Wang, D., Jordan, M. & Rich, N. (2000) Survival after emergency department thoracotomy: review of published data from the past 25 years. *Journal of the American College of Surgeons* **190** (3), 288–98.

Scottish Intercollegiate Guidelines Network (SIGN) (2000) *Early Management of Patients with Head Injury*. Available online at: www.sign.ac.uk/guidelines/fulltext/46/index.html.

Out-of-Hospital Resuscitation

Ben King

17

INTRODUCTION

Since ancient times attempts have been made to revive casualties collapsing in the community and for centuries investigators have striven to find the most effective treatments. In the last 100 years, the rise in heart disease in the industrialised nations has led to it becoming the commonest cause of cardiac arrest in the pre-hospital setting. This chapter sets out the background to current guidelines and explains the evidence that has led to their adoption. It particularly considers the development of pre-hospital defibrillation as a vital contribution to community resuscitation. Finally, there is discussion on developments that may improve survival in the future.

AIMS

This chapter discusses how out-of-hospital resuscitation has changed in line with the nature of sudden death.

LEARNING OUTCOMES

At the end of the chapter, the learner will be able to:

❑ identify *causes* of out-of-hospital cardiac arrests;
❑ describe *factors that influence survival*;
❑ discuss *out-of-hospital basic life support* (BLS) and *advanced life support* (ALS);
❑ identify why out-of-hospital resuscitation sometimes *fails to happen*;
❑ outline the development of *out-of-hospital defibrillation* and *community-based defibrillators*;
❑ discuss whether out-of-hospital resuscitation is *worthwhile*;
❑ discuss possible *developments in the future*.

OUT-OF-HOSPITAL ARRESTS

It is estimated that 12 000 cardiac arrests take place in the United Kingdom (UK) each year in public places (Department of Health (DH) 2000). Cardiac disease accounts for more than 50% of out-of-hospital cardiac arrests and death is usually caused by a lethal tachyarrhythmia, which in turn is usually precipitated by acute coronary syndromes (ACS; Rosen *et al*. 2001). Tachyarrhythmias are fast unstable heart rhythms which may also be caused by electrolyte imbalance, drug toxicity and cardiomyopathies though these are much less common (Engdahl *et al*. 2002). For the remainder of this chapter, acute coronary syndrome will assume to be the cause of out-of-hospital arrest.

The true incidence of cardiac arrests presenting with ventricular fibrillation (VF) is unknown; however, available data suggest that it is over 80% (Norris 1998). It is also known that the chances of successfully defibrillating the patient fall by between 7 and 10% per minute if defibrillation is delayed (Resuscitation Council UK 2005).

Survival is greater amongst patients who suffer their arrest in public places rather than at home; however in one UK study, 80% of instances of ALS provided by paramedics were in the casualty's home (Dowie *et al*. 2003).

Predictors of likely survival of cardiac arrest (Engdahl *et al*. 2002)

Short-term survival
- Witnessed arrest;
- Bystander cardiopulmonary resuscitation (CPR) performed;
- VF first recorded rhythm.

Long-term survival
- Arrest caused by acute myocardial infarction (AMI);
- Patient of moderate age;
- Good heart function post-event.

OUT-OF-HOSPITAL BLS
Research since the 1960s has consistently confirmed that CPR is a vital holding manoeuvre to perfuse the heart and brain with oxygen, though it rarely itself restores circulation. The start of CPR in the community setting preceded out-of-hospital defibrillation, so the benefit of this holding manoeuvre would have been limited.

Further research has confirmed the hypothesis that CPR plays another important role in prolonging the period of VF before deterioration into asystole (Holmberg *et al*. 2000). In one study, shockable rhythms were present in 48% of witnessed out-of-hospital arrests where bystander CPR was being performed and in only 27% of cases where it was not (Dowie *et al*. 2003).

As discussed in the Chain of Survival (see Chapter 5), the question has arisen as to whether the lone rescuer should phone first or commence CPR. When the arrest is likely to be cardiac in origin, the lone rescuer should phone first prior to starting CPR. Healthcare professionals should be competent in performing CPR and should understand the rationale for seeking help first.

Dilemmas in out-of-hospital resuscitation
Despite advances in training and wider public awareness, members of the public fail to initiate CPR for many reasons.

Lack of training

The bystander may fail to initiate resuscitation due to:

- no previous training;
- fear of making things worse;
- panic;
- fear that they may perform CPR inadequately.

Those communities where a high proportion of the population are trained to perform CPR have demonstrated higher survival rates (Eisenberg *et al.* 1990). Training will reduce the rescuer's fear of making things worse and also bolster their confidence to respond appropriately.

Compression-only CPR

Despite the risk of infection-transmission being low (Resuscitation Council UK 2005), many people who attend CPR training express reluctance to perform mouth-to-mouth ventilation, particularly on strangers.

In the situation where the rescuer is reluctant to perform mouth-to-mouth ventilation, chest compressions alone offer significant improvement over nothing at all. The benefit to the casualty will be further enhanced if the airway can be opened to allow the compressions to generate some tidal volume. Compression-only CPR is also used when emergency medical dispatchers provide instruction to untrained rescuers performing CPR for the first time (Resuscitation Council UK 2005).

Several studies have suggested that if bystanders perform CPR it may be just as effective for them to perform compressions only rather than full CPR incorporating mouth to mouth (Bohm *et al.* 2007, Iwami *et al.* 2007, Nagao 2007). The benefits to this approach not only remove the reluctance of performing mouth to mouth, but also mean a significantly greater number of compressions that will be performed per minute without gaps for ventilation. In light of this, the American Heart Association (AHA) has changed its recommendations to compression-only CPR for lay people or for those who lack confidence to perform CPR (AHA 2008).

The European Resuscitation Council and the Resuscitation Council (UK) in contrast have decided to retain the recommendation for CPR as in the 2005 guidelines (Soar & Nolan 2008).

OUT-OF-HOSPITAL ALS

Early defibrillation offers enormous benefit to the casualty of out-of-hospital arrest for two reasons. Firstly, it is known that these patients are in a shockable rhythm most of the time. Secondly, it is this group of pre-hospital arrest patients who are most likely to survive (Cummins *et al.* 1985). Sudden cardiac death frequently happens to those with no previous history of heart disease and two-thirds of deaths from coronary artery disease occur in the community (Engdahl *et al.* 2002). If an AMI patient suffers a cardiac arrest in the presence of a paramedic, he or she has a 40% or greater chance of survival to discharge (Norris 1998).

Out-of-hospital defibrillation

Until pioneering work in Belfast (Pantridge & Geddes 1967), the only place a defibrillator would be found was in a hospital. Even if effective CPR was provided delaying advanced interventions reduced survival because:

- simple CPR (without oxygen, drugs or airway management devices) can only stave off hypoxic brain damage for a limited time;
- it will not offer any protection of the airway so it is likely that stomach contents will be aspirated into the lungs;
- CPR will delay the process of VF fading away to asystole but will not prevent it.

Pantridge and his team converted a hospital mains defibrillator to run on two car batteries which was then carried in an ambulance. This equipment, weighing 70 kg, allowed defibrillation en-route to hospital and was occasionally manhandled into patients' houses (Pantridge 1989).

Training out-of-hospital personnel in the necessary skills of rhythm recognition and defibrillation has continued in many countries to allow them to perform unsupervised defibrillation. This has become standard practice to such an extent that it is difficult to believe that it was not always viewed this way.

Defibrillators in the community

The National Service Framework for Coronary Heart Disease states that:

> People with symptoms of a possible heart attack should receive help from an individual equipped with and appropriately trained in the use of a defibrillator within 8 minutes of calling for help, to maximise the benefits of resuscitation should it be necessary. (DH 2000; 27)

Automated defibrillators have allowed defibrillation to be performed by those with no rhythm interpretation skills. Defibrillator technology alongside developments in batteries has allowed units to become smaller and lighter to the extremely portable machines seen today.

A number of creative strategies have made use of these developments.

- British general practitioners – in one study, when GPs reached the scene with a defibrillator within 4 minutes, 90% of patients were in a shockable rhythm and 70% survived to hospital; 60% of those patients were discharged alive. One in 20 MI patients attended by a GP, arrests in the doctor's presence (DH 1999).
- Casino security guards – security guards at Las Vegas casinos were given training in the use of automated external defibrillators (AEDs). When the first shock was delivered within 3 minutes, the survival rate to discharge was 74% (Valenzuela *et al*. 2000).
- Untrained bystander defibrillation – three airports in Chicago put defibrillators in public places. Over a period of two years, 21 casualties were treated and 18 were in VF. Of these 18, 10 were free of neurological impairment 12 months after the arrest. Six of the survivors were successfully defibrillated by persons with neither training nor experience of using an AED (Caffrey 2002).

First responder schemes

First responder schemes are joint initiatives between the ambulance service and voluntary members of the public who are provided with resuscitation training and equipment. They are called at the time the ambulance controller puts out the 999 call and may reach the casualty first, speeding up time to the delivery of the first shock.

Public access defibrillation

As stated earlier in the chapter, most arrests happen in the casualty's own home, which has led some authors to suggest putting defibrillators in the homes of at-risk individuals who could be defibrillated by their family members (Eisenberg 2001).

IS OUT-OF-HOSPITAL RESUSCITATION WORTHWHILE?

Some investigators have looked at the quality of life experienced by those who survive a cardiac arrest in the community. In terms purely of outcome, those who survive to hospital discharge have an 88% chance of living for one year and a 75% chance of five-year survival (Kuilman *et al.* 1999).

For some casualties, being left with long-term damage may be a worse outcome than dying. What is deemed an acceptable quality of life will vary between individuals.

One investigator who looked at how survivors viewed their own quality of life studied 50 survivors from out-of-hospital arrest and compared their quality of life against a control group. There were reduced scores for physical mobility and energy levels amongst the survivor's group but factors such as anxiety, depression and general well-being were the same. Perhaps the most important statistic was that 49 out of 50 arrest survivors felt that their lives were 'worth living' (Saner *et al.* 2002).

In a small-scale study where very rapid defibrillation and impressive survival were achieved, all the survivors left hospital able to care for themselves, suggesting they did not suffer severe neurological dysfunction (Valenzuela *et al.* 2000).

DEVELOPMENTS FOR THE FUTURE

Challenges to improving survival from cardiac arrest in the community include the following.

Training

Cities such as Seattle, where a high proportion of the public have received training in CPR, show the impact this can make on survival (Cummins *et al.* 1991). The challenge for future programmes is to train significantly more people whilst encouraging those who have previously been trained to return for annual updates. Other ways to deliver training are being explored, including replacing the instructor with a video. This system of group self-instruction has, in some studies, shown significant improvement over instructor-led classes (Woollard 2003).

Compression-only CPR for lay public may enhance numbers trained and give greater confidence for them to respond in an emergency.

Earlier defibrillation

As increasing numbers of defibrillators arrive in the community through initiatives such as first responder and public access defibrillation schemes, it is likely that the time taken to the first shock will lessen (Davies 2002). Greater access means greater chance of a defibrillator arriving prior to the arrest and the shock being delivered in the early phase of VF. At the time of publication, there are in excess of 6000 defibrillators across the UK in out-of-hospital locations (British Heart Foundation 2008).

Smarter defibrillators

Defibrillators are now smaller and cheaper than ever before to the point where families of high-risk patients may purchase them. Waveform analysis employed in newer machines allows the rhythm to be analysed during chest compressions as the software filters out the artefact of compressions.

Advisory defibrillators currently inform the operator when a shock is appropriate. In the future, the machine may also be able to analyse the rhythm while chest compressions are ongoing, thus improving perfusion to the vital organs.

There is ongoing study into the benefits of performing CPR before defibrillation in unwitnessed arrests. This is due to the risk of shocking the patient's heart into asystole if they have had some time without CPR. Waveform analysis allows some units to look at the rhythm to predict whether the shock should be delivered immediately or after a period of CPR. The voice prompts of the machine can then advise the operator to the appropriate action.

Thrombolysis

Thrombolytic therapy has been shown to improve survival in individual case studies but larger studies have yet to prove their benefit (Baubin 2001). A major study to evaluate the benefit of thrombolysis in out-of-hospital cardiac arrests is ongoing (Bottiger 2005).

REVIEW OF LEARNING

❑ Cardiac disease accounts for more than 50% of out-of-hospital arrests.
❑ CPR is an important holding procedure, though lack of training and reluctance to perform mouth-to-mouth ventilation may inhibit CPR delivery.
❑ Early defibrillation offers enormous benefit to the out-of-hospital arrest casualty.

CONCLUSION

Out-of-hospital cardiac arrest is an important issue due to the prevalence of cardiovascular disease in the industrialised nations, added to the fact that one-third of those suffering an AMI will die before reaching hospital. Research has clearly demonstrated that steps such as calling for help and simple BLS can have a huge impact on successful recovery. When early defibrillation is also achieved, success rates are improved still further. As increasing numbers of defibrillators appear in out-of-hospital settings, healthcare professionals must become aware of the contribution that these simple steps can make.

REFERENCES

AHA (2008) Hands-only (compression-only) cardiopulmonary resuscitation: a call to action for bystanders to adults who experience out-of-hospital sudden cardiac arrest: A Science Advisory for the Public from the American Heart Association Emergency Cardiovascular Care Committee. *Circulation* **117**, 2162–7.

Baubin, M. (2001) Recombinant tissue plasminogen activator during cardiopulmonary resuscitation in 108 patients with out of hospital cardiac arrest. *Resuscitation* **50**, 71–6.

Bohm, K., Rosenqvist, M., Herlitz, J., Hollenberg, J. & Svensson L. (2007) Survival is similar after standard treatment and chest compression only in out-of hospital bystander cardiopulmonary resuscitation. *Circulation* **116**, 2894–6.

Bottiger, B.W. (2005) International multi centre trial protocol to assess the efficacy and safety of tenecteplase during cardiopulmonary resuscitation in patients with out of hospital cardiac arrest: the Thrombolysis in Cardiac Arrest (TROICA) Study. *European Journal of Clinical Investigation* **35** (5):315–23.

British Heart Foundation (2008) *Beating Heart Disease Together*. Available online at: www.bhf.org.uk/ research_health_professionals/non-research_grants/defibrillators.aspx. Updated 31 January 2007.

Caffrey, S.L. (2002) Public use of automated external defibrillators. *New England Journal of Medicine* **347**, 1242–7.

Cummins, R.O., Eisenberg, M.S. & Hallstrom, A.P. (1985) Survival from out-of-hospital cardiac arrest with early initiation of CPR. *Annals of Emergency Medicine* **3**, 114–18.

Cummins, R.O., Ornato, J., Theis, W. & Pepe, P. (1991) Improving survival from sudden cardiac arrest: the chain of survival concept. *Circulation* **83**, 1832–47.

Davies, C.S. (2002) Defibrillators in public places: the introduction of a national scheme for public access defibrillation in England. *Resuscitation* **52**, 13–21.

Department of Health (1999) *Saving Lives: Our Healthier Nation*. Department of Health, London.

Department of Health (2000) *National Service Framework for Coronary Heart Disease*. Department of Health, London.

Dowie, R., Campbell, H., Donohoe, R. & Clarke, P. (2003) 'Event tree' analysis of out of hospital cardiac arrest data: confirming the importance of bystander CPR. *Resuscitation* **56**, 173–81.

Eisenberg, M.S. (2001) Review article – cardiac resuscitation. *New England Journal of Medicine* **344**, 1304–13.

Eisenberg, M.S., Horwood, B.T., Cummins, R.O., Reynolds-Haetle, R. & Hearne, T.R. (1990) Cardiac arrest and resuscitation: a tale of 29 cities. *Annals of Emergency Medicine* **19**, 179–86.

Engdahl, J., Holmberg, M., Karlson, B.W., Luepker, R. & Herlitz, J. (2002) The epidemiology of out-of-hospital 'sudden' cardiac arrest. *Resuscitation* **52**, 235–45.

Holmberg, M., Holmberg, S. & Herlitz, J. (2000) Effect of bystander CPR in out-of-hospital cardiac arrest patients in Sweden. *Resuscitation* **47**, 59–70.

Iwami, T., Kawamura, T., Hiraide, A. *et al.* (2007) Effectiveness of bystander-initiated cardiac-only resuscitation for patients with out-of-hospital cardiac arrest. *Circulation* **116**, 2900–7.

Kuilman, M., Bleeker, J., Hartman, J. & Simoons, M. (1999) Long-term survival after out-of hospital cardiac arrest: an 8 year follow-up. *Resuscitation* **41**, 25–31.

Nagao, KftS-Ksg (2007) Cardiopulmonary resuscitation by bystanders with chest compression only (SOS-Kanto): an observational study. *Lancet* **369**, 920–6.

Norris, R.M., for the UK Heart Attack Study Collaborative Group (1998) Fatality outside hospital from acute coronary events in three British health districts. *BMJ* **316**, 1065–70.

Pantridge, F. (1989) *An Unquiet Life – Memoirs of a Physician and Cardiologist*. Greystone Books, Belfast, Northern Ireland.

Pantridge, J.F. & Geddes, J.S. (1967) A mobile intensive care unit in the management of myocardial infarction. *Lancet* **2** (7510), 271–3.

Resuscitation Council UK (2005) *Advanced Life Support Course Provider Manual*, 4th edn. Resuscitation Council UK, London.

Rosen, K.R., Sinz, E.H. & Castro, J. (2001) Basic and advanced life support and acute resuscitation and cardiopulmonary resuscitation. *Current Opinion in Anaesthesiology* **14**, 177–84.

Saner, H., Rodriguez, B., Kummer-Bangerter, A., Schuppel, R. & von Planta, M. (2002) Quality of life in long term survivors from out-of-hospital cardiac arrest. *Resuscitation* **53**, 7–13.

Soar, J. & Nolan, J.P. (2008) Cardiopulmonary resuscitation for out of hospital arrest. *BMJ* **336** (7648), 782–3.

Valenzuela, T.D., Roe, D., Nichol, G., Clark, L., Spaite, D. & Hardman, R. (2000) Outcome of rapid defibrillation by security officers after cardiac arrest in casinos. *New England Journal of Medicine* **343**, 1242–7.

Woollard, M. (2003) Less teaching means more learning. *Heartstart* (British Heart Foundation), Issue 16, 4–5.

Index